THE WINNING WELLNESS METHOD

DISCOVER THE HIDDEN GUIDE TO WEIGHT LOSS AND HEALING YOUR BODY WITHOUT TRADITIONAL YO-YO DIETING

DR. AUSTIN WIN

Copyright Notice © 2017 Winning Wellness & Physical Therapy, LLC
All rights reserved.

No part of this publication may be reproduced, distributed, or transmitted in any form or by any means, including photocopying, recording, or other electronic or mechanical methods, without the prior written consent of the author.

CONTENTS

Dedication vii
Foreword ix
Acknowledgements.. xi
Introduction... xiii

Chapter 1   The Winning Wake Up Call................................... 1
Chapter 2   The Winning Formula 11
Chapter 3   The Food Breakdown... 20
Chapter 4   Nutrition & Injury Recovery 60
Chapter 5   Operation Dream Team.. 72
Chapter 6   Kitchen Friendly Cooking 78
Chapter 7   The Winning Secrets... 95
Chapter 8   Operation Fountain of Youth............................. 102
Chapter 9   Mastering Mindfulness....................................... 108
Chapter 10 Injured to In Shape 115

FAQs.. 125
Free Healthy Gifts... 137
References 139
About the Author 141

DEDICATION

To my father and mother for all their love and sacrifices. To my professors and mentors who ignited my passion for nutrition and physical therapy. To all the experts I've met in my life who helped me become the person I am today. To all my friends, family and loved ones who believe and support me. To all my clients and patients who have inspired me to make the world a better place by impacting even more lives. You all are what drives me today.

FOREWORD

I've known Austin Win for quite a few years and one of the things that marveled me about him is his ability to have such an expertise in the nutritional aspect of taking care of your body during the rehabilitation process. The fact that Austin has been able to combine both of them together is groundbreaking! This is something that has been needed in the rehabilitation industry for many years. I am so thankful to Austin for moving forward with his mission of getting clients in the rehab world the tools they need to have a complete recovery through addressing nutrition as part of their rehabilitation plan. I totally 100% endorse Austin and his endeavors. Well done.

Greg Todd
Creator of Smart Success PT Online Academy
Co-owner of Renewal Rehabilitation
President of Physical Therapy Builder

ACKNOWLEDGEMENTS

My thanks and gratitude go out to all the wonderful people I've encountered in my life that I have been able to positively impact. You all have helped me become the person that I am today. This includes all of my personal training clients, all of my customers in the restaurant and most importantly all of my patients in the hospital and PT clinics.

I also want to give a special thanks to all those who believed in me and inspired me to write this book so I can give massive value to the world. Thank you Greg Todd and Paul Gough for all of the amazing support with the communities you have built. None of this would have ever been possible without you both and I am truly grateful.

Finally, I would like to acknowledge with gratitude the love and support from my soul mate, Shelli. Thank you for your unconditional love and unbelievable support you have given me. You continue to inspire me to be the best version of myself and I can't thank you enough for going on this journey with me!

INTRODUCTION

I'd like to start this book off by giving you some information on what typically goes on in the United States. About a third of the country are obese and many people do not exercise.[3] And when people try to get into the habit of healthy eating and exercise they dive into extreme diets and lifestyle changes that are in no way, shape or form sustainable. Sound familiar? In today's world many people are taking advice from those with no educational background or degree in nutrition which makes it extremely difficult knowing what to do or eat for your health. When's the last time you've gone online without hearing about the latest diet, nutrition trend, magical pill or supplement?

Health statistics show that over 133 million Americans suffer from at least one chronic disease, and that number continues to grow.[15] What's worse is that most of these conditions can be prevented with good nutrition and exercise, especially when working with a qualified health professional. Now imagine when the typical overweight or obese individual becomes injured. Do you think that life just now got easier or harder for them?

It now makes it much more difficult for them to recover from their injury (depending on the severity), lose weight and keep it off in the long-term. Instead of using nature's healing power in the form of good food and nutrition, many people will resort to pills, injections, surgery or painkillers. Worst of all, many people believe it is normal. That's the way it is and nobody can be blamed. People naturally look for the easiest way out and the easiest solution with the least amount of effort involved. If so many people have a difficult time losing weight on their own, can you imagine how painful it will be to attempt to lose weight when they're injured and in physical therapy?

This book is for people who suffer from unhealthy eating habits, crash dieting, and setbacks due to an injury. Losing weight during this time may seem almost impossible to do with everything you have going on in the moment, but I am here to tell you that there is a way and it is possible. Let me tell you what I have typically seen during my career as a Registered Dietitian and a Physical Therapist. A patient, call her Mary, is overweight and has been dealing with right knee pain for quite some time. Mary does not eat healthy at all, nor exercises as part of her lifestyle. Mary just thinks that the nagging right knee pain and ache will miraculously go away if she just keeps on doing what she's doing during the day. Mary believes that the knee pain will magically disappear by praying and hoping, while at the same time not really doing anything specifically to help her right knee out.

And so, Mary waits and waits until the knee pain becomes so severe that she can no longer walk because of the excruciating pain. That's about the time when she decides she really needs to look further into the situation and figure out what's going on. Mary goes to the doctor and then gets told she has severe arthritis and will need to get a right knee replacement. Mary is now in tons of fear because she is afraid of having surgery and does not want to undergo any operation. The doctor recommended her physical therapy and so she decides to start the rehab with the hopes of avoiding surgery altogether.

To Mary's surprise her right knee actually starts to feel better a few weeks into physical therapy, but at this point she still has not changed any of her habits or lifestyle. Despite the right knee getting better, she then starts to notice that her left knee is giving her problems also. So, what does Mary do? She takes painkillers because it's the easiest thing she can do to relieve her pain. The problem is that she starts taking them over and over again every single day.

Without realizing it she becomes easily addicted to the painkillers and starts to have other medical issues. She is now depressed because she now has both knees to worry about. Mary follows up with her doctor and now has been told that she may need two knee replacements, which will result in her having to continue physical therapy even longer.

In her best-case scenario, she continues with physical therapy and goes through with the surgery for both of her knees. That process can take well over a year to recover. Although she has agreed with the doctor's recommendations, she still has been unable to lose any weight throughout this whole time. The good thing is that now her knees don't bother her anymore, but the bad thing is that she is now starting to feel more pain in her lower back. This is a vicious cycle and I would not want anyone else to experience what Mary had to go through, but unfortunately it happens all the time.

Mary has been under lots of stress and has been experiencing increased pain throughout her joints due to the amount of extra weight and pressure on her body. Mary is just one example of the type of patients I have seen who have come in for physical therapy. There are others as well who I've seen with much smaller injuries and others with much more severe injuries. The point is that if you are overweight or obese and have become injured, now is a good time as any to start taking charge of your life and change your habits. Losing weight, especially under the guidance of a qualified Registered Dietitian, can help you reduce the risk of knee osteoarthritis and other related problems.[11]

This is the reason why I wrote this book. I understand how difficult this journey can be, especially if you are facing a life crisis. Dealing with an injury and learning about nutrition to lose weight can be very daunting, but I'm here to tell you that it is not. It can be if you let it, but I want to show you how you can lose weight and feel great without going on a crazy diet. Working professionals, students, and many others who struggle with their nutrition during an injury have already experienced great success implementing the tips and advice found in this book.

The goal of this book is not to give you a specific diet to follow, but to give you principles and practical information you can use throughout the rest of your life. I want to set you up for success and not failure. I've witnessed countless people who have participated in several diets throughout their lifetime to only lose weight fast and quickly gain it right back. If you are looking for another quick fix and strict diet to follow then this may not be the book for you. There are many dangers of dieting, which all include negatively impacting your body's metabolism, increasing the risk of eating disorders, heart disease and loss of muscle tissue, bone density, and other detrimental side effects.

My goal is to have you start losing weight in an entirely different approach. Yes, you will have to include and exclude certain foods when you have a certain medical condition or are injured, but this is not about following a specific diet. Also, please do not think of this as an encyclopedia of nutrition. Yes, you will learn about nutrition, but think of this as your road map. This book is for those who finally want to lose weight and keep it off without going on a restrictive diet. As you move forward with this book please know that knowledge alone is not power. Execution is. The action you take upon it is far more important than the information you learn from it.

The information and recommendations given here are not based off theory. Everything is based off the exact methods that have helped thousands of people throughout the globe. This book was written to help guide you on the path towards better health and wellness when injured. There is such a vast amount of information on the internet that it can be difficult to truly decipher what information is correct and what is not. This book was written to give you more clarity. If you follow the advice given in this book you will be 10x more confident in achieving your goals than you currently do now.

My goal is to provide you with quality information so that you can feel confident and not overwhelmed when making decisions for your health. The advice given in this book is not intended for you to take extreme measures, which unfortunately is what cause many people to give up. The advice given in this book is geared towards you taking a practical approach to your health that can last you a lifetime. There are no revolutionary techniques given in this book, just simple guidelines and reliable information from a specialist. I can't make any big or bold guarantees without knowing your medical history, but I can tell you that after reading this book you will have much more clarity on what your next steps to take are.

Now get ready to discover the hidden guide to weight loss and healing your body without traditional yo-yo dieting!

CHAPTER 1
THE WINNING WAKE UP CALL

I really want to explain the importance of mindset first. This is going to be a long process and a lot of difficulties and obstacles may come up if you're injured and trying to lose weight.

You may have heard that in order to lose weight it's 80% nutrition and 20% exercise. Although that is true what I believe to be even more accurate is that in order to lose weight it is 80% mindset and 20% nutrition. The secret sauce will not primarily be a how problem, but it will be a what problem. So instead of asking the how questions such as "How do I lose weight?" I want you to start asking the what questions, which will ultimately build your foundation for success. You'll find out what I'm talking about in a minute. If this part isn't done then nothing else I tell you matters, just as how the 2nd or 3rd story of a house won't matter if I haven't built the ground floor first.

I really want to emphasize the importance of your mindset and how you should really just stay passionate to your goals and really know your WHY. I will say this a few times throughout the book because the reason is to really ingrain it in your head so that when your motivation runs low your WHY will be your fuel to reignite your passion and drive you to continue moving forward. My WHY is my family. I appreciate life so much and I'm very thankful for each day that I am alive. I take nothing for granted. When I think of my health I also think about how my nonexistence will impact others in my life. I want to be around my family and friends as long as I can so that I will continue to positively impact their lives. Now I know I will be unable to do all of those things if I don't have my health first and that is why I use that as my fuel. You must focus on what you can control and the decisions you make today will impact your health for the better or worse. Now what is your WHY?

Consistency is key. It doesn't matter how good or "bad" you ate in one day. What matters most is how you consistently eat throughout the week and months. We all have our good days and our bad days. What determines our future is how well we bounce back from the bad days and continue to strive to achieve our goals no matter how many obstacles come in the way or how many "excuses" we want to give ourselves. Nobody said this would be easy, but that's why it is so important to have the right mindset first. Think about progress, not perfection.

Most people attempt to achieve perfection and give up when things get tough because they could not make their days and weeks perfect. Please let me remind you that a journey of a thousand miles begins with one step. All you need to do is continue to step in the right direction.

The only limitations you have are the ones you set up in your own mind.

THE POWER OF QUESTIONS

Most people have a difficult time achieving what they want because they simply do not ask themselves the right questions. Asking the right questions will force you to think and come up with the right answer to the actual problem. Below is a list of 10 questions I highly recommend you to start asking yourself as you begin this weight loss journey.

1. What are my goals?
2. What do I believe I can achieve in order to reach my goals?
3. What am I willing to give up in order to reach my goals?
4. What do I have to change in order to achieve the results I'm looking for?
5. What motivates me? (Know your WHY)
6. What do I think of myself? What is my self-image?
7. What are my bad habits?
8. What thoughts run through my head? What kind of negative things do I tell myself?

9. What stresses me out?
10. What support do I have? Or what kind of people do I surround myself with?

Now write down the answers to the questions above before you move on. This is important! Please do not skip any steps. Answering the questions will help bring more awareness to your life and guide you down to the path of success. By knowing the answers and writing them down you now have a starting framework and direction to go. I'm going to take some time and explain why knowing the answers to each question is vital.

You need to know your goals, both long term and short term. If you don't know what your goals are how do you know if you will achieve them? Second of all, do you really believe that you can achieve your goals? Believing that you can actually achieve your goals is much more important than having goals in mind. Anyone can dream and have goals, but do they really believe they can achieve them? That's a massive difference because if you do believe in your ability to achieve your goals you will make the necessary actions to do so. What things are you doing right now that you know you can sacrifice in order to achieve your goals? If you aren't willing to make a change or give things up to reach your goals then no changes will happen and you have to accept that.

You also need to know what motivates you and the reason why you're doing all of this in the first place. Dig deep down within yourself and find your WHY. Having a list of things that motivate you will really help you out, especially on the days when you feel like giving up.

In addition, having a list of your bad habits will bring more awareness to yourself on things to be conscientious of. You now can avoid certain bad habits because you now realize and accept what they are. In other words, you need to know what to change in order to change them. You must also be careful of the story you tell yourself because the story can become a reality by just constantly thinking about it. What you think of yourself is crucial and having a positive self-image may be difficult, but it is necessary to massively impact the quality of your life. Therefore, knowing the thoughts that run through your head and the negative things that you tell yourself will give you a chance to change them.

Stress is necessary in people's lives in order for them to grow. Simply put, when you exercise your body you are inducing stress on it so that your muscles can become stronger and grow. Everybody deals with certain stressors during their life, but the big difference is on how they react to the stress. Too much stress on your body can have a detrimental effect on your health and make it much harder for you to lose weight. So, by knowing what stresses you out, you also give yourself a chance to change how you react and think about the stress. For example, two different people can undergo the same stress and have an entirely different outcome or reaction to it. Person A can be stressed and eat chocolate cake to make her feel better while person B can receive the same stress and instead take a nice long walk outside. Same stress, two different outcomes.

Lastly, the support you have or don't have will play a crucial part in your weight loss journey. Have you heard that you are the average of the five people you spend most of your time with? Well if everyone you hang around with are not as motivated as you are to make a change and will not give you the necessary encouragement you need to succeed, then it will seriously be much more difficult for you to reach your own health goals. Without a support system you will either fail or have to be extremely disciplined and relentless towards achieving your goals so that nothing will stop you from obtaining what you want. Having support and guidance can have a profound difference in your life.

Now after answering the 10 questions above I want you to review questions 1-5 daily.

This will help you stay on track and not lose focus. What would it feel like if you achieved your goals? How would life look like? Can you see yourself being that person? Keep that in mind and use your answers to motivate you. For questions 6-10 I want you to analyze your answers and start figuring out ways that you can change them to help you achieve your goals. For example: If you tell yourself "I am overweight and I can never lose weight" - change that to "I am beautiful, in control of my body and can lose any weight I desire". If one of your bad habits is to drink soda with every meal try substituting it with drinking water instead. If you negatively tell yourself "This is hard and there's no hope for me" change that to "I know this is not easy, but it will be worth it and I can do this". If an injury or your situation stresses you out and in return triggers you to respond negatively to it, think of other areas in your life that you can be grateful for. Think of other ways to change your reaction to the stress. If you are surrounded by people who will not help take you to the next level then change that by joining a community of like-minded people in similar situations. Whatever your answers are try finding ways to change them for the better.

SELF-ASSESSMENT

Now it's time for the self-assessment. This is the time for you to be honest with yourself and get a baseline measurement of where you are starting today. It's important for me to say that this is in no way, shape or form as thorough as getting a nutrition consultation by a Registered Dietitian (which I highly recommend), but for starters this will work. This is meant to bring you more awareness on areas that you are lacking and can improve on. Remember, this is only the beginning and your answers will change as the weeks go by. Here are some things to start thinking about:

1. What are your current eating patterns?
2. Do you plan out your meals for the day?
3. Do you currently cook?
4. How often do you eat out in a week?
5. How much water do you drink in a day?
6. Do you exercise? If so, how many times per week and for how long?
7. What are your sleeping patterns?
8. What are your stress patterns?
9. How much fruits and vegetables do you eat in a day?
10. What are you grateful for? What makes you happy?

These are all thought joggers to get your mind going before officially taking the self-assessment.

As you ask yourself these questions you automatically open a loop in your brain to start to come up with some solutions to these problems. All I'm doing right now is bringing more awareness to your life. Now take a few minutes to complete the assessment below.

Please rate yourself from 1-5 on the statements below (1 = poor, 5 = excellent)

1. I eat at regular times each day and rarely skip meals
2. I plan my meals and snacks ahead of time
3. I take my time to eat my meals (at least 20 min) without distractions (TV)
4. Most of my meals are cooked at home
5. I set short term goals for myself and review them weekly
6. I drink at least eight glasses of water a day
7. I include some kind of exercise into my schedule each day
8. I eat at least five servings of fruits and vegetables each day
9. I do resistance training at least 2-3 times per week
10. I get 8 hours of sleep daily
11. I incorporate de-stressing activities daily
12. I feel in control with my life and balance it well with no stress
13. I shop from a prepared shopping list and only buy items on the list
14. I read food labels carefully in detail
15. I feel in control of my diet and my body
16. I am confident in my abilities to change to reach my goals
17. I know my goals and why they are important to me
18. I minimize eating high-fat foods like desserts, fried foods, pastries, and sauces
19. I rarely dine out during the week, unless for special occasions
20. I am able to dine out and stay very consistent with my goals

Now add up the total number and that will be your score. What did you think of your self-assessment? Did you score a 100? If you did then you most likely do not need my help because the majority of the population will definitely not score a 100. Remember, this is progress and not perfection. You now know what areas you are weaker on and can start working towards to improve your scores. Don't try to improve everything all at one time. Focus on the biggest 3-5 things that will make the biggest change for you. Based off the self-assessment, if you only had five moves in order to turn your goals into reality what would they be? Write them down right now before you move on. The rest can wait.

Next, we are going to get some quick and easy objective information. I want you to record the following information and take some pictures of yourself. You will take pictures from three different angles: the front, the back and the side. The reason for doing this is for you to have a starting point and not ever forget how far you have come. Look back at these as you make some wins with this book.

We easily get caught up thinking about the future and strive to reach one goal after another, that we actually never really look back to see how far we have come. It's important to realize your mini successes and be grateful for every milestone you have achieved. Now save these pictures because you will use them to inspire yourself and others with your future transformation.

Dr. Austin Win

Height: _____

Weight: _____

Calculate BMI:

Equation: Weight (lbs)/ Height (in)^2 x 703

Example: 185 lbs/ (65 in)^2 x 703 = 30.8 (obese)

Please mark your BMI on Chart

BMI Chart

BMI < 18.50	**Underweight**
BMI < 16.00	Severe Thinness
BMI 16.00 - 16.99	Moderate Thinness
BMI 17.00 - 18.49	Mild Thinness
BMI 18.50 - 24.99	**Normal Weight**
BMI 18.50 - 22.99	Lower Range
BMI 23.00 - 24.99	Upper Range
BMI 25.00 - 29.99	**Overweight / Pre-Obese**
BMI 25.00 - 27.49	Lower Range
BMI 27.50 - 29.99	Upper Range
BMI ≥ 30	**Obese**
BMI 30.00 - 34.99	Obese Class I
BMI 35.00 - 39.99	Obese Class II
BMI ≥ 40.00	Obese Class III

Once again recording these objective measurements such as your weight and your BMI does not tell the whole story, but it gives you a starting point. Don't be discouraged. Use this information and compare it to the goals you have written for yourself earlier. You now have a framework for goal setting. You know where you are at this point and the journey you have to go through in order to reach your goals. Don't let your goals scare you. Say them out loud with confidence on a daily basis and be definite in your goals. You will achieve them. I believe in you! To print this self-assessment go to www.drwinsecrets.com and get it now.

CHANGE YOUR THOUGHTS, CHANGE YOUR LIFE

Okay now that you have taken your self-assessment you know exactly what areas you are lacking on and where you should place your focus towards during the next few weeks. I want to take this moment to talk about your thoughts and comfort zone. Your thoughts are the basis for everything and what you believe to be true, or not to be true, will be correct in your eyes. Our comfort zones is in the subconscious mind and it holds all of our beliefs, values and habits. So, we take action regularly upon what is in that zone on a daily basis. I want to debunk some myths and raise awareness to some things that may have gone in your comfort zone and been "programmed" in your head for a long time. Think of a computer and how you will drag and drop items into the trash box. That is essentially what we will be doing together so that you can unravel the misinformation and create a new comfort zone, which ironically will be uncomfortable since you are doing something new. But in order to change we must be willing to step outside our comfort zone to create new habits and lifestyle changes.

Here are some myths that you need to be aware of:

1. Carbohydrates are bad
2. It's normal to feel aches and pain as we age
3. In order to lose weight, I need to starve
4. In order to lose weight, I have to avoid all of my favorite foods
5. I should lose the weight first, and then exercise
6. Exercise is about no pain, no gain
7. I have to go on a special diet to lose weight like a ketogenic diet

8. Diet soda will keep me thin
9. All calories are created equally
10. Losing weight is fast and easy
11. There are secret foods to instantly burn body fat
12. You should avoid all sugar- even fruit
13. Being slim means that you are healthy
14. High fat foods are bad for you
15. All you need to do is detox and drink a shake

Your comfort zone will be tested greatly over time and old habits will find a way of coming back, you just need to be aware of them! That is why small changes over time last the longest. Be aware of your own self-talk and old comfort zone messages that will get you to fall back to what it believes is the right messages. Some examples are "It's okay I will just skip today and start tomorrow", or "This is too hard, I will never lose weight". If you give into these messages and fall back to these old habits for a couple of weeks, the chances of you succeeding are slim. What will be the big hitter for you is your focus, your discipline, and consistency. So be comfortable with being uncomfortable so that you can maintain your new healthy habits.

Now before you move on to the next chapter I would like you to take a minute and go back to your goals. Look at it and then close your eyes and envision the person you want to become. Think about how you want to look like and how that will make you feel. Think back to your WHY! Remember it and ingrain it within your heart and mind because that will be your biggest motivator and reminder to why you are doing what you're doing right now.

TAKE ACTION: SEND ME AN EMAIL

It's time to put your foot down, draw a line in the sand, right here, right now and get some real accountability. Email me right now (my email is Austin@drwinsecrets.com) with the subject line "I've Put my Foot Down" and tell me that you are committed to Winning in your Wellness. And tell me that you will do what it takes to once and for all get your health back. I want to know if you are all in on this. Please email me if you are committed. Let's do this!

CHAPTER 2
THE WINNING FORMULA

Congratulations on making it to the next chapter. We have just gone through your goals, questions to ask yourself, the self-assessment and debunked some nutrition myths. Remember what I said about celebrating the small wins? Yay! Give yourself a pat on the back. As you continue to progress further into the book you will learn exactly why the nutrition myths I've listed are not facts. I will start this chapter off by first talking about calories and energy needs. In order to lose weight, you must first understand how it works and that is why I'm giving you the formula.

Your health is determined by how many nutrients you eat in your total amount of calories you intake. A calorie is just a unit of energy and the energy value that we apply to foods. Your calories come from your macronutrients, which we will talk about in the next chapter. Nutrients on the other hand are found in vitamins, minerals, fibers and naturally occurring plant chemicals called phytochemicals. In order to lose weight, you must focus on eating foods with higher amounts of nutrients in relation to calories, or in other words nutrient dense foods. The amount of calories you need depend on several factors such as your age, gender, height, weight, activity level and stress factor (as if you're injured).

I'm not a big fan of calculating calories and having someone pull out their app or calculator every time they eat, but for some people it works. Therefore, I will briefly explain some numbers to both maintain weight and lose weight. If your calories or food energy is balanced, meaning the amount of calories you're eating and expending are equal, then you have weight maintenance. 3,500 calories = 1 pound. So, if you eat 3,500 calories in a day and expend 3,500 calories in a day you have achieved energy balance. The equations I will give you are by no means the most accurate, but it will give you baseline information to work with. For more in depth and accurate numbers I recommend you seek out a Registered Dietitian to help you with your individualized needs. Go to coach.drwinsecrets.com to find one now.

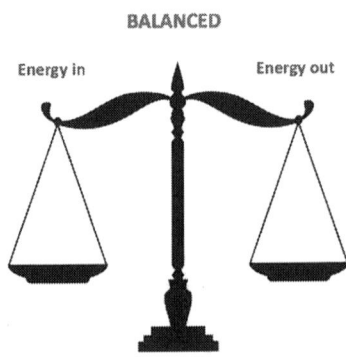

To calculate your maintenance calories: Body weight in lbs. x 12

In order to lose weight, you must expend more energy than you intake. So, if you start eating higher amounts of nutrient dense foods (less calories) and start exercising more (burning calories) you will be able to lose weight. You need to be in a calorie deficit.[4] Here is a visual below.

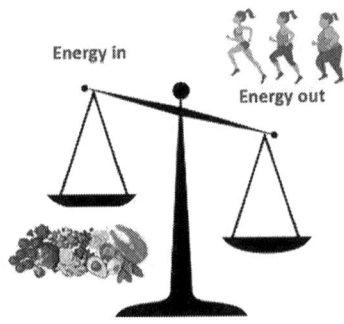

To calculate your weight loss calories: Body weight in lbs. x 10

The Winning Wellness Method

What you do not want to do is go in the opposite direction and gain weight, which is where most people are. Understanding weight gain is an easier concept for people to comprehend because many people have experienced it themselves.

If you overeat, or have an excess of calories, and do not exercise (expend energy) you will surely gain weight. You are consuming more calories than you are burning and the weight scale will show. Here is another visual below.

Weight Gain

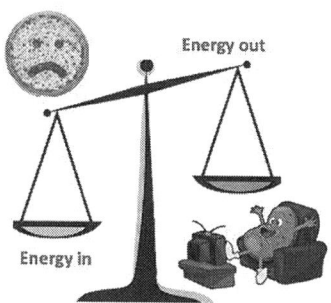

Be aware of empty calories. Empty calories are foods that provide you no nutritional benefit. Therefore, you need to eat foods that are high in nutrients so you don't consume too many empty calories. Eating foods that are high in fiber, low in calories and rich in nutrients will fill you up and prevent you from overeating. I will give you the food breakdown in the next chapter so you know exactly what foods I am talking about.

Science shows us that the more nutrients and fiber you have the less hungry you will become and therefore are less likely to overeat. Aim for natural whole foods and disregard any advertised weight loss pills or injections you see on late night television.

You now have a basic understanding of calories. The secret to losing weight and keeping it off is to eat large amounts of high-nutrient foods. Others may say that the quickest way to lose weight is to put the fork down! I'm here to give you practical advice that you can take action on and sustain. If there is any diet to follow I recommend you follow the winning diet.

What is the winning diet you ask? It is a "diet" or way of eating that works for you. It is a lifestyle eating pattern that you can sustain in the long term and WIN in to have permanent weight control without feeling deprived or entirely giving up your favorite foods. This is perfect for those who have been on diets in the past and it has never worked out for them. You must commit yourself to eating in a way where you can have high nutrient foods at least 80% of the time. Leave the other 20% for your favorite foods.

CHANGE YOUR HABITS CHANGE YOUR LIFE

Changing your eating patterns is difficult, but it is not impossible. You must have faith. Many people have emotional connections to food and have built a deep connection or even addiction to the American diet. After reading this book you will have a clear understanding of how to achieve the results you are looking for. You will know how to reach your goals even faster without any doubts. This may be a book that you will have to reference and go back to, or even reread to truly master the concepts. The most important factor is that you stay committed and take action to reach your goals, no matter how long it takes.

Here are 10 simple tips to help you lose weight:

1. Choose energy dense foods
2. Think nutrients and add color to your meals
3. Eat frequent meals
4. Eat slower
5. Plan ahead and cook
6. Drink plenty of water throughout the day
7. Carry healthy snacks
8. Be consistent
9. Stay balanced
10. Stay committed

Now I want to revisit a question and have you take some time to reflect upon it. What bad habits increase your calories? What things do you do during the week that increase your calories? Or what things do you not do to stop yourself from eating too many calories? Take some time to write that down. After you have figured those things out the next thing you have to do is figure out WHY.

Is it a lack of:

- Self-control?
- Information?
- Time?
- Exercise?
- Planning?
- Skill?
- Confidence?
- Support system?
- Belief?
- Self-worth?
- Value in health?
- Desire to change?

After you have figured out WHY or the cause of the habits you can then come up with a solution for it. For example, if you know that you have a bad habit of eating out every day and the WHY for it is a lack of planning you can now fix it. You now have a chance to change that bad habit because you've brought a specific problem to your awareness that you can improve on.

Now prioritize the list with your biggest three bad habits you can start working on to change.

Your list may be constantly reviewed and reprioritized as your habits change. You can do this on a weekly basis to reflect on your habits. To summarize calories and weight loss it all relates to your energy balance.

Energy out > Energy in = Weight Loss
Energy in > Energy out = Weight Gain
Energy in = Energy out = Weight Maintenance

Remember 3,500 calories = 1 lb. So, if you eat 500 fewer calories or burn 500 calories a day for 7 days you will lose 1 lb. in a week. So, what can you do to reduce the amount of calories you are currently having? What bad habits can you change? What one habit, that if you do it consistently will make a positive and drastic impact on your weight? If you've realized so far, I have not spoken much about numbers, but have been teaching about concepts and principles.

For the calorie counters you can easily use the formulas I've given in this chapter to calculate your weight loss calories.

To calculate your weight loss calories: Body weight in lbs. x 10

For example: You weigh 200 pounds. Using the formula above 200 x 10 = 2,000 calories. You need to consume approximately 2,000 calories a day to start losing weight. This can be tracked by apps such as Lose It or MyFitnessPal, but it is not absolutely necessary.

Numerous people have been able to lose weight by simply food journaling and using other tools I give you throughout this book. Make it a simple habit to start food journaling for at least 21 days. Small positive changes done consistently over time can have a great impact on your health. You will be amazed at the results when you do this.

Now it's time to take action! Before you move onto the next chapter you must figure out your winning formula. What things can you do today to start eating healthier? What foods can you start adding in your life so that you can continue to eat that way and stay healthy? What are some ways that you can eat healthy and consistently until it feels just normal? The concept of weight loss is simple, but the actions and steps it takes to achieve weight loss may not be.

Everyone has their own winning formula. Finding out what routines or habits you can personally change and sustain in the long term to achieve permanent weight loss will be crucial. What is your winning formula? Do you need to stop drinking soda, eating chips, burgers and fries every week? Do you need to include more veggies with your meals? Do you need to food journal? Write your answers down!

FOOD CONTRACT

Now that we have discussed calories, habits and weight loss I want you to take what you have learned so far and apply it. Below on the next page shows a sample food contract that is between you and yourself.

You can download it at www.drwinsecrets.com or write it down on a sheet of paper and place it key areas such as next to your bed, work desk and refrigerator to be constantly aware of your goals.

Write 3 short term goals for this week: (What, how, when, where)

Example: I will not drink any soda this week and instead I'll drink water by carrying a bottle with me everywhere

1.
2.
3.

Give yourself accountability! Give each day a ✘ or ✔

Goal	Mon	Tues	Weds	Thurs	Fri	Sat	Sun

Identify barriers to completing your goals and how you will overcome them:

_____

_____

_____

_____

Reward: (Pick a non-food reward)
Example: I will treat myself to the spa if I have achieved all of my goals I have set for the week

_____

_____

_____

Sign: _____   Date: _____

TAKE ACTION: IT'S APPLICATION TIME

Step 1: Answer the following questions:

    I. What things can I do today to start eating healthier?

    II. What foods can I start adding in my "diet" consistently?

    III. What is my winning formula?

Step 2: Complete the Food Contract. To print this out go to www.drwinsecrets.com and download it now.

Step 3: Send me a selfie!

    Yes I want to see proof that you completed the homework. If you're serious about this, then take a selfie of yourself with the book right now and get ready to make yourself accountable. Trust me I know this may feel a bit uncomfortable doing, but I'm telling you this small action will make a world of a difference. So go and take that book selfie!

    Next, if you're on Instagram go on there right now and post this picture up using the #winningwellness and tag me @draustinwin so that

I know you actually did it! Remember that knowledge alone is not power, it's the actions taken from the knowledge. If you're not on Instagram then email your selfie to me. Let's take action and have fun in the process! Email me at Austin@drwinsecrets.com

CHAPTER 3
THE FOOD BREAKDOWN

This chapter is all about breaking food down into understandable components so you know how food can work for you. In order to make some real specific changes you must first understand what impact certain foods have on your health and what your foods are composed of. We'll be going over carbohydrates, fiber, fats, protein, hydration, sugar, micronutrients and portion control. Lastly, we'll come up with an action plan!

First let's discuss carbohydrates since that appears to be one of the most talked about subjects. Your first thought may be to think that in order to lose weight you have avoid all carbs, when in fact that is not true.

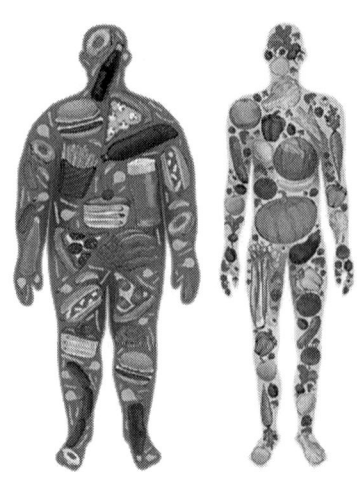

Yes, in America most people eat too many highly processed carbohydrates and as a result do gain weight, but remember it all boils down to your total amount of calories. Let's go over what carbs are, what they do to your body and how to choose them wisely.

The picture above is a simple visual of how food can impact your body. Both of their diets are mostly composed of carbohydrates so the kind of carbohydrates you eat matter. If your diet is mostly composed of pizza, burgers, donuts and other highly processed carbs then your body will react in such a way. On the other hand, if your diet is mostly composed of

The Winning Wellness Method

high-nutrient carbs, you automatically are eating less calories, more fiber and getting much more nutritional benefits.

Let's start off with what carbs are. It is your body's main source of energy. Your brain uses carbs, specifically glucose. Your muscles even use carbs for energy! If you go for a run or sprint as if you're getting chased by a dog your body will be using carbs to fuel your energy.

Carbs is one of the three macronutrients (other two are fat and protein), meaning it is required in large amounts in the body. There are two types of carbs called simple and complex carbs. Let's begin with the simple carbs, which is what most people in America consume way too much.

Think of simple carbs as all of your sweets and treats. They are loaded with sugar!

Simple carbs get digested really fast and also increase your blood sugar really fast. It is an easy way to spike glucose in your body and store more fat around your belly. They lack real nutrients.

Simple carbs include food items such as candy, juice, jam, syrup, soda, sugar, frosting and all your other sweets. Simple carbs definitely should be eaten wisely. You should not be eating them all the time. You can leave your sweet tooth cravings for the 20% of your meals. The problem is that most people are almost addicted to these carbs that they eat it on a daily basis.

To give a scientific explanation, when you eat these carbs it causes a rapid increase in your blood sugar which will trigger the hormone insulin to drive the sugar out of the blood and into your cells. As a result, too much insulin promotes more storage of body fat.

Eventually when your blood sugar or glucose levels get too high in your blood, your body will continue to pump out insulin in attempt to lower your blood sugar. The problem is that eventually your body will become resistant to insulin and you will continue to put on more body fat. To make things worse you will still crave more food due to the lack of nutrients in these simple refined carbs and gain more weight. You do not want to get to the point where your body becomes insulin resistant. A lot of factors go into play for that to happen, but if you do become insulin resistant you will have a whole host of problems including delayed wound healing. Now that doesn't help if you're trying to recover from an injury.

Complex carbohydrates are everything else that is not simple! Think of your starchy foods, fruits and veggies. They take a long time to digest and have a slower release of energy. As opposed to simple carbs, complex carbs gradually increase your blood sugar levels. They include items such as bread, rice, potato, banana, apples, oatmeal, beans, peas, pasta, lentils, and other fruits and vegetables. Most people in America consume an excess of low nutrient carbohydrates such as white bread, white rice, white flour, white potatoes, and pasta. When choosing carbs decide what will give you the most amount of nutrients with the least calories.

Whole grains, fruits and vegetables should be the bulk of the diet. When choosing carbs there are some things to consider. Think about nutrients, portion sizes, food tolerance and digestion around activity. For example, it may not be a good idea to eat lots of fiber right before you have some physical activity. Actual whole grains have more nutritional value, higher fiber and take a longer time to digest when compared to white products.

Dietary guidelines recommend you to eat approximately 50% of your calories from carbohydrates. An easy way to go about this is to recognize your portion sizes and to not go over your servings of starchy carbohydrates for each meal. Load half your plate with fruits and vegetables or eat as many as you want because they are low calorie high fiber nutrient dense foods. You are mostly counting the starchy carbohydrates such as potatoes and rice.

When losing weight ask yourself "What's the least amount of carbs I can eat in a meal and still be satisfied?" Once again for the calorie counters here are some numbers and ideas to work with below. Carbohydrates provide 4 calories per gram of carb.

For 2,000 calorie diet eat up to 4 servings of carbs per meal
For 1600-1800 calorie diet eat up to 3 servings of carbs per meal
For 1200-1500 calorie diet eat up to 2 servings of carbs per meal

So how much exactly is a serving of a carb? 1 serving of a carb = 15 grams of carbs.

- 1 slice bread (1 oz)
- ¼ large bagel
- 1 small fruit

- 1/3 cup cooked pasta
- ¼ large baked potato
- 1 tbsp. jelly
- 1 tortilla (6 inch)
- 1 cup milk
- 1/3 cup cooked rice

So, from this list if you decide to eat 1 cup of rice that is equivalent to 3 servings of carbs.

Any more than that you will be on the verge of going over your calories for the meal. This is just a general rule of thumb. This by no means is set in stone. Remember what matters most at the end of the day is how many total calories you consume, but if you stay consistent with the eating patterns it will make it much easier to reach those goals.

Counting carbohydrates becomes very important when you have diabetes or are insulin resistant. I do not wish anyone to have this common disease. What I do wish is that you are more aware of the type of carbohydrates you eat and the quality of the carbohydrates you consume.

Remember that carbs are the primary source of energy and fuel. You want to recognize the differences between simple and complex carbs. Choose carbs wisely and make whole grains, fruits and vegetables the bulk of your carbohydrate diet. Save the sweets for the 20% portion of your favorite foods. Stick to your portions and count carbs as needed. One simple trick to decrease your cravings of eating too many carbs in a meal is to eat them last. Try it out.

Drink water, eat your protein and fats first, then eat your carbs. Eat slowly! You may realize that you did not need to eat as many carbs as you originally thought. Don't be afraid to leave them behind and throw them away if you can't finish them either. The compounding effect of this simple trick can go a long way for your weight.

WHAT ARE THE GOOD FATS TO EAT?

Another macronutrient and major energy source is fats. Simply put, good fats keep your heart healthy while bad fats can damage your heart and increase the risk of disease. So, there are essential and non-essential fats. We'll focus on the essential ones because that's what your body needs to get from foods because it can't produce it on its own. Fats help you absorb nutrients, specifically vitamins A, D, E and K which are considered fat soluble. Fats are important and necessary for brain protection and function. They also help protect your organs and support cellular growth. We cannot survive without fats so going on a complete fat-free diet is not a good idea.

Dietary guidelines suggest that you consume about 30% of your calories from fats. Keep in mind that fats are your most concentrated source of calories. It is more than twice the amount of calories/gram when compared to carbs and protein. They provide 9 calories per gram of fat.

An example is one tablespoon of oil = 120 calories. Now how much broccoli would you have to eat to get 120 calories vs ingesting one tablespoon of oil? That's the difference. So, you must definitely watch your portion sizes for these kind of fats.

A quick and easy way to estimate your portions for these fats are to use your thumb!

Serving size: 1 Teaspoon = Thumb Tip = 45 calories
Use thumb tip for items such as:
Oil
Butter
Mayonnaise

Serving size: 1 Tablespoon = Thumb = 120 calories
Use thumb for items such as:
Peanut butter
Salad Dressing
Sour Cream

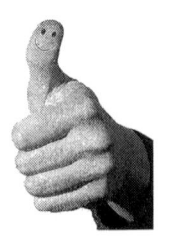

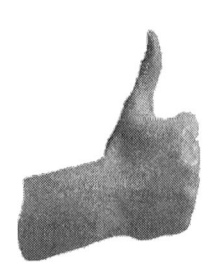

Once again, your body cannot produce essential fats on its own, which is why it's called essential fats. They must be obtained from the diet. It includes Omega-3 and Omega-6 fatty acids. Omega-3 fatty acids have been known to provide many health benefits including protective effects of the heart and brain. They are considered anti-inflammatory in nature and cold-water fish is the best source. Many fatty fish are good for us to eat. They have tons of protein and good fat. Those good fishes should be eaten at least twice a week. Some examples include salmon, herring, whitefish, cod, mackerel, sardines, canned light tuna and anchovies.

Some fish are better if you just eat them once a week due to the mercury content, which is another subject. Those fish include white canned albacore tuna, pompano, grouper, snapper, and mahi mahi. Now the fishes that I definitely do not recommend to eat are tilefish, swordfish, shark and king mackerel because they have the highest level of mercury.

There are also plant-based sources of Omega 3's that I recommend, which contain ALA. Some examples include flaxseed, hemp seed, chia seeds, walnuts and brussel sprouts.

Although they are not as a reliable source of EPA and DHA which are found in fish, they do provide a lot of nutritional benefit so I recommend eating both. What matters most is that you create a way to include those foods into your diet.

Omega 6 fatty acids are considered pro inflammatory, which have the opposite effects of Omega 3's. They are found mostly in processed vegetable oils with the highest amounts in sunflower oil, corn oil, soybean oil, and cottonseed oil. Your body needs a healthy balance of Omega 3's and Omega 6, so you want to limit the amount of Omega 6 that you eat because an excess of it will contribute to more inflammation in your body. The majority of people don't need any more inflammation in their body so eating additional Omega 6's will only further trigger the release of pro-inflammatory chemicals. Below is a visual breakdown of dietary fats.

Comparison of Dietary Fats

DIETARY FAT	SATURATED FAT	LINOLEIC ACID (omega-6)	ALPHA-LINOLENIC ACID (omega-3)	OLEIC ACID (omega-9)
Canola oil	7	21	11	61
Safflower oil	8	14	1	77
Flaxseed oil	9	16	57	18
Sunflower oil	12	71	1	16
Corn oil	13	57	1	29
Olive oil	15	9	1	75
Soybean oil	15	54	8	23
Peanut oil	19	33	*	48
Cottonseed oil	27	54	*	19
Lard	43	9	1	47
Palm oil	51	10	*	39
Butter	68	3	1	28
Coconut oil	91	2		7

*Trace. Fatty acid content normalized to 100%.

The above chart breaks down all the oils in percentages of saturated fat, Omega 3's, Omega 6's and monounsaturated fats. Continuing on with our discussion, you can see the dietary fats with the color blue indicating the percentage of Omega 6 fatty acids. We will now differentiate between the good fats, the bad fats and the dangerous fats that you should be aware of. Not all fats are of equal value and you will soon be able to distinguish the differences.

The good fats are the unsaturated fats and they come primarily from plant-based foods. Unsaturated fats are liquid at room temperature and they can lower your cholesterol levels. Some examples are avocado, olive oil, canola oil, nuts, seeds, fish and fish oil.

Bad fats include saturated fats that can raise your blood cholesterol levels. You want to limit the amount of saturated fats that you have in your diet, which should be approximately 5% of your calories. Who actually measures that anyway? Most people don't so I want to give you some practical advice to practice. Limit saturated fats such as lard, fatty beef, skin on poultry and palm oil as much as you can to reduce the overall intake of the bad fats. If you noticed from the chart above coconut oil is also included in the category of saturated fats. Coconut oil is a special type of oil with medicinal properties, but it still does include calories and saturated fats so it should not be seen as a magical solution to all of your problems. It should be used wisely and with careful attention. Don't add it into everything you eat or drink.

The dangerous fats are the trans fats that raise your risk of heart disease. Trans fats have the ability to raise your blood cholesterol levels and negatively impact your health. These foods should be avoided or eaten with much more caution and awareness. Partially hydrogenated oils, fried foods, donuts, biscuits, cakes, margarine and frozen pizza all contain trans fats. Yes, you may be thinking to yourself, but who doesn't like to eat donuts? I'm not saying to absolutely not eat it, just donut give up! Be aware of the harm these foods can have on your health, especially when consumed frequently. Satisfy your cravings with these foods once in a blue moon or on special occasions like your 90th birthday.

The healthy fats that you should include in your diet are olive oil, canola oil, avocado, avocado oil, nuts, seeds, nut butters, fish, fish oil and coconut oil (in moderation). You want to choose high-quality healthy fats which include your Omega-3s and unsaturated fats. Have less saturated fats, Omega 6 fatty acids and severely limit trans fats in your diet. Watch your portion sizes with fats and start thinking of ways where you can add more healthy fats to your meals.

These fats may help keep you satiated longer and reduce your risk of heart disease.

WHAT ARE THE BENEFITS OF PROTEIN?

The last macronutrient that is needed in large amounts in your body is protein. Protein has several functions in the body, but one of its main roles is to help you build and maintain your muscle mass. Eating more protein can help keep you full and burn more body fat because of a term called diet-induced thermogenesis. This thermic effect of food is basically the energy production process the body will go through when metabolizing food. It has been shown that eating higher protein foods will induce more weight loss and satiety when compared to a low protein diet.

Protein is not a good source of energy, but it is necessary for muscle recovery. Diving into some science, amino acids are the building blocks of protein. There are essential and nonessential amino acids. The essential ones must be consumed from your diet because the body cannot make it on its own. The non-essential amino acids are much less important because the body can make it on its own and therefore it doesn't need to be received from foods. So, what is a high-quality protein source you ask? Meat, fish, eggs and milk have all the essential amino acids.

Most plant proteins are considered incomplete proteins because they are missing an essential amino acid. Combining foods such as your grains and beans can provide a complete protein source. You can experience health problems if your diet is too low in essential amino acids. While it is important to include healthy fats and higher fiber foods into your diet, you must also include lean protein in as well. Some examples are chicken breast, turkey breast, lean ground beef, top round steak, fish, seafood, pork tenderloin, eggs, low-fat dairy, beans, peas and lentils.

The amount of protein that you need in your body is dependent on several factors such as your age, gender, activity levels or stress factors. It is suggested that you eat at least 20% of your calories from protein, but optimally it should be higher. On average you should have a total daily protein intake of 1g/kg of body weight. This number can be as high as 1g/lb. of body weight if you're an athlete or experiencing recovery from a major surgery. One easy way to be consistent with your protein intake is to stay calm and look at your palm!

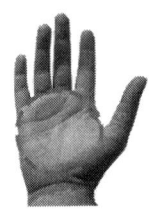

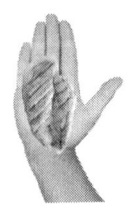

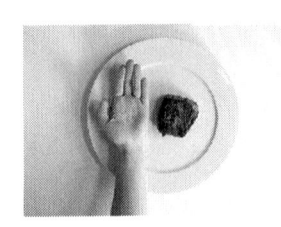

Protein provides 4 calories per gram of protein. 1 oz of cooked meat is approximately 7 grams of protein. So, for example if you had 3 oz of baked chicken you would have consumed approximately 21 grams of protein. This is a good way to estimate the amount of protein you're eating if you're calculating or you can just use your palm. The frequency and times when you eat your protein is important as well. Ideally you would like to consume a consistent amount in every meal, but there may be times where you'll be unable to for some reason. The goal is to have an even distribution throughout the day.

Aim to eat protein at every meal. If you're unable to then you should definitely make sure you eat a higher protein breakfast and consume more protein right after exercising. Eating a higher protein breakfast will make sure you start your day off with more protein in your body.

Also, consuming protein after exercising or doing physical therapy will help rebuild those muscles you were working on. Another trick to guarantee you get your protein in during a meal is to eat the protein first. That way you will have insured you've eaten all the protein, even if you got full and could not finish your plate.

Some examples of high protein foods that provide 20 to 30 grams of protein are 4 oz lean meats (fish, chicken, beef, turkey), 2 whole eggs and 2 egg whites, 1 can of tuna, 1 can of salmon, and 1 scoop of protein powder. Some protein snack ideas are Greek yogurt, hummus, peanut butter, hard-boiled eggs, low-fat milk, beef jerky, cottage cheese, and protein bars. Good sources of vegetable protein include broccoli, peas, beans, lentils, tofu, tempeh, edamame, chia seeds, hempseeds, soy milk, sweet potatoes, quinoa and whole grains.

Protein variety is king. You must not avoid protein in your diet because you need it to build and keep your muscles strong. It is a myth that eating too much protein will impair your kidney function.[12] Stay lean with protein and remember all your high-quality protein sources. Keep calm and look at your palm when it comes to portioning animal sources of protein. Eat larger portions of your vegetable proteins like your green super healthy foods as that will be the key to your success of permanent weight loss. Aim for even protein portions throughout the day and time them around your physical activity. For example, you may want to consume a nutritious blueberry protein shake with chia seeds right after your exercise session.

SHOULD I BE EATING MORE FIBER?

Fiber is essential to your health and the majority of people do not include enough of it in their life. There are two types of fiber, soluble and insoluble fiber, and both should be incorporated into your diet. Oats are an example of soluble fiber. They help lower your cholesterol, decrease your blood sugar levels, keep you fuller longer and help you lose weight.

Think about the times when you have had oatmeal in the morning. The oats blend with the water and create a thick consistency afterwards. That is essentially what is happening in your digestive tract. The soluble fiber is forming a gel like solution to bind up the cholesterol and blood sugars to promote a healthy gut. Other foods containing soluble fiber include beans, legumes, flax seeds, and fruits such as apples and bananas.

Insoluble fiber is also good to promote a healthy digestive system. It includes foods such as your whole grains, fruits, vegetables, nuts, seeds and wheat bran. Insoluble fiber helps promote more movement through your digestive system to make sure you don't have problems such as constipation. Unfortunately, constipation can be the least of your worries if your diet has been deficient in fiber for a very long time. Other health problems such as diabetes and diverticulitis can occur from having too little fiber in your life. The average person should consume about 20-30 grams of fiber a day at a minimum. You can meet this need by eating five servings of a variety of fruits and vegetables in a day. Try and aim for a higher fiber goal.

You can get large amounts of fiber in your diet when you include more plant-based foods such as fruits, vegetables and beans. Fiber will help control the rate of digestion and slow down the blood sugar absorption in your body. It will also reduce your cravings because the fiber from the plant-based foods will fill you up. I must warn you though. If you are going to now start including more fiber in your diet and it hasn't been a big part of your life before you must start slow. If not, you will increase your chances of stomach aches and pains with more frequent visits to the bathroom. Drink more water and eat more fiber at a gradual pace. A good rule of thumb to remember is to make sure you go number two at least once a day.

Eating higher fiber natural foods will reduce your chances of chronic diseases such as diabetes and cancer, while at the same time lowering your waistline. In order to lose weight, you need to make it a priority to include higher fiber foods into your life. The people who do that are the healthiest. Simply make it a habit to substitute low fiber foods such as your white rice, white bread and pasta with other natural foods that have not had their fiber removed. Doing this often will naturally "cleanse" your colon and give you significant health benefits. You must train your taste to slim your waist!

WHY IS HYDRATION IMPORTANT?

Now after speaking about fiber hydration couldn't be more of a perfect segue. Your body is made up of 60% water so your body depends on water to survive. Proper hydration is just as important as making proper food choices. You want to drink water early and drink regularly, especially as you increase the amount of fiber in your diet. If not, you will become constipated and have a really hard time in the bathroom, no pun intended. Water is the most essential nutrient and your body needs water to function.

Most people do not drink enough water and may be dehydrated without realizing it. Lack of hydration can affect you both mentally and physically. Some signs of dehydration include dry mouth, dark yellow urine, peeing very little, muscle cramps, fatigue, headache, dry skin and confusion. You are at an even greater risk of dehydration if you live in a hot climate. Some simple hydration tips include carrying a water bottle or hydro flask with you at all times, drinking water with every meal, setting reminders, checking your pee color, and drinking early and regularly. Look at the hydration urine chart below. You're at risk for cramping or a heat illness once you reach number 4. The symptoms become worse once you pass that and the color of your urine becomes darker. Ideally you would want to have a pale-yellow urine color. Stay hydrated!

Hydration Urine Chart

- 1-3 = Hydrated
- 4-6 = Dehydrated
- 7-8 = Severe Dehydration

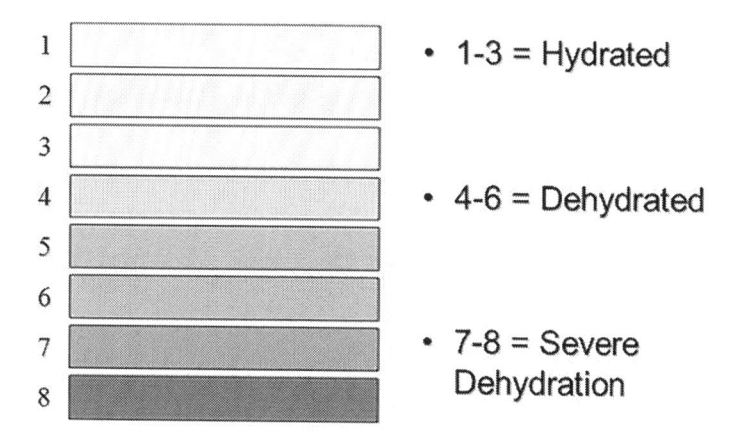

You can lose weight by simply drinking enough water. You often times may think that you're hungry when in fact your body just needs more water! One simple trick to determine this is that when you're eating and think that you're still hungry, drink a large glass of water and wait a few minutes. If after waiting you feel that you weren't as hungry as you thought then congratulations! You were just thirsty and you saved yourself some calories. Drinking water before meals can also save you from eating more calories than you may need.

So how much water should you have in a day? One simple estimation is to drink half of your body weight in ounces. For example, Mary weighs 200 lbs. 200 lbs. x ½ = 100 ounces of water. Mary needs 100 oz of H20 or 12.5 cups in a day (8 oz = 1 cup. 100 oz/ 8 oz =12.5 cups).

If you know how much water you should drink in a day it will give you a goal to reach as you sip water regularly throughout the day. Do not overdrink! There is such a thing as over-hydration.

Once again this is just a simple estimation, but for a more accurate assessment I recommend speaking with a Registered Dietitian. Go to coach.drwinsecrets.com to find one now.

Hydration becomes especially important when you are exercising. You want to drink to replace the amount of water that was lost. More specifically, you want to drink two cups of water for every 1 pound lost when exercising. Plain water can keep you hydrated during exercise. You want to drink before, during and after your exercise training sessions. Make that a good habit. A question that is asked often is if you should have a sports drink when exercising. That is typically recommended only when performing higher intensity exercises that are lasting greater than 1 hour. Otherwise drinking water is sufficient. So please remember to drink early and drink regularly. You can check to see how you are doing with your hydration when you check your pee color. Is your pee a light-yellow transparent color or does it look like the color of a highlighter? Use the chart to check your pee color often to make sure you are staying on track.

CHOOSE NUTRIENT-RICH FOODS

Micronutrients are needed in your body in just small amounts, but they're really important to maintain your normal body function. This includes both vitamins and minerals that are essential to life. Going deep into depth and detail about each vitamin and mineral is really out of scope for this book, but I want you to really understand that you have to think in terms of nutrients. That is what is most important! So, think about nutrients whenever you eat. Variety is king and that means you want to eat a variety of foods to get the most health benefit. That's why it's so important to have a variety of colors on your plate and eat a good combination of foods. I will give several examples below of why this is crucial.

Starting off with Vitamin C, it is a powerful antioxidant that can prevent free-radical damage that contributes to aging and other aging related diseases. It one of my favorite vitamins because of how many significant roles it plays. It is important to include in your diet to boost your immune system, handle all physical stress, mental stress, repair tissues in your body and help maintain your collagen that is found in your hair, skin, and nails. You'll learn more about collagen later, but it is just a protein that supports many body structures. You can find Vitamin C in foods such as strawberries, cantaloupe, pineapple, oranges, brussel sprouts, broccoli, kale, sweet peppers, guava, collards, cauliflower, papaya, spinach and cabbage.

I'm sure you've heard of B vitamins, which help provide you energy by converting your food into fuel. You can mostly find them in your whole grains (wheat, rice, rye, oats) and fortified cereals. They are also found in green leafy vegetables. Most of the B vitamins are removed when the grains are highly refined, which is why it's important to consume whole grains.

Vitamin D can be obtained naturally from the sun and it is most important for maintaining your bone density. Vitamin D will help you keep your bones strong and retain the calcium and phosphorus in your body.

Maintaining your bone density and reducing unfortunate events such as a hip fracture is vital to maintaining your longevity. You can prevent fractures and falls with adequate levels of Vitamin D. Once again you can receive Vitamin D directly from the sunlight by going outside 10-15 minutes a day or by obtaining it from foods such as egg yolks, fortified milk, or fatty saltwater fish (tuna, cod, herring, halibut).

Vitamin A is good for your vision and maintaining good healthy skin. It plays an important role in the immune system and it is essential for the proper function of your eye. It is found in high amounts in in fish liver oil from cod, salmon and halibut. The vitamin A precursor, beta carotene, is found in yellow-orange fruits and vegetables such as carrots, cantaloupe, apricots, parsley, spinach, kale, and turnip greens.

Vitamin E has antioxidant powers that enhances resistance to disease and helps with prevention of aging-related degenerative diseases. It aids in red blood cell formation and may slow the aging process by protecting the body from free radicals. It also plays a role in wound healing and reducing scar formation that is commonly found after surgery. There have been studies showing people with osteoarthritis benefiting from Vitamin E supplementation with reduced joint pain and inflammation.[9] Some food sources include wheat germ oil and unprocessed vegetable oils such as safflower oil. Smaller amounts can be found in spinach, whole grains, nuts, and legumes.

Vitamin K has a role in maintaining healthy bones, hearts and having healthy blood clothing. Low levels of vitamin K have also been associated with osteoporosis and fractures.

Vitamin K can be found in a variety of foods with the highest amounts in dark green leafy vegetables such as spinach, collard greens, turnip greens, kale, broccoli and swiss chard.

These green vegetables have a powerful effect on reducing the incidence of hip fractures. If you're currently on certain medications such as blood thinners I recommend you speak with a Registered Dietitian before increasing the amount of these foods in your diet.

There are several minerals that exist, but once again the point of all this is to make you aware of how important it is to include a variety of high-nutrient foods in your diet. It is out of the scope of this book to go into depth of every single mineral that is out there, but I will mention a few major ones. Starting off with calcium, it has many vital functions throughout the body including maintaining strong, healthy bones. If someone is deficient in calcium over a long period of time they will be at an increased risk for fractures, even when doing something as simple as sneezing.

Osteoporosis affects millions of Americans especially over the age of 50 and it is a common problem that can be caused by inadequate calcium intake. There are other functions of calcium including the contraction and relaxation of muscles, including the heart. The richest food sources are in milk and dairy products such as yogurt and cheese. Other foods providing calcium include seafood (shrimp, clams, oysters), canned sardines, canned salmon, and green leafy vegetables such as kale, collard greens, mustard greens and turnip greens.

If you consume a lot of soft drinks you can deplete the calcium levels in your body. The reason being is that soda contains higher amounts of phosphorus and you want to maintain an even ratio of calcium to phosphorus. In other words, you should consume at least the same amount of calcium as you do phosphorus. The more soda you drink, the more phosphorus you intake, and the more it will impair your absorption of calcium and therefore it will decrease your bone density over time. Also, don't forget the amount of calories you're consuming and the more weight you are putting on by simply drinking soda. It's another recipe for increased pain and weight gain.

Magnesium is required for strong healthy teeth and bones. Approximately 60% of the United States is at risk for magnesium deficiency. One of magnesium's major roles is to maintain the proper function of nerves and help your muscles relax. Having a high occurrence of muscle spasms can be related to magnesium deficiency. Osteoporosis has also been related to poor magnesium intake just like calcium. Can you now see why it's so important to include a variety of foods in your diet? You can find magnesium in high amounts in almonds, pumpkin seeds, whole grains, halibut and soybeans.

Potassium is another mineral that is also used for muscle contraction and nerve transmission. Potassium deficiency symptoms may include nausea, muscle weakness, muscle spasms and cramps. Potassium can become depleted in your body after severe tissue injury due to surgery. Good food sources of potassium include dairy products, sweet potato, bananas, beans, legumes, clams, fish, spinach and poultry. Sodium is another important mineral that must exist in balance with potassium in the body. Most people consume way too much sodium and as a result have high blood pressure and other related diseases. Your sodium intake becomes very important as you get older and you want to keep it at a minimum. Leave the saltshaker on the table and do your best to watch out for high-sodium foods including canned good, sausages, bacon, luncheon meats and frozen foods. It is recommended to consume less than 2,300 mg of sodium in one day, which is equivalent to about 1 teaspoon of salt!

The goal of this section was to emphasize the importance of having high nutrients foods in your diet because of the amount of vitamins and minerals they include. You have just learned the benefit that these macronutrients have in your body and how they can be found in a wide variety of foods. Don't be overwhelmed and don't undergo analysis paralysis. Intelligibly create a plan and figure out how you can make this work for you. Do not overthink this. Plainly think how you can add more color to your life, literally. With all of this information, what I really want you to do is ask yourself certain questions whenever you're about to eat. You can ask yourself the following:

1. "Are there any nutrients in these foods?"
2. "Am I getting any nutritional benefit from eating this?"
3. "Does my plate look colorful?"
4. "Do I have a variety of different foods on my plate?"
5. If not, "How can I make this meal healthier?"
6. "How will this food help me?" (More energy? Weight loss? Feel better?)

Asking yourself some of these questions prior to eating will force you to eat more nutritious foods in order to get the benefit of these micronutrients. You are now bringing more awareness to yourself that consuming more of these energy dense foods will have a massive impact to your health and weight. If you fail to plan then you must plan to fail. Once again think of progress, not perfection. Small changes over time yield big results.

IS IT OKAY TO EAT SUGAR?

You don't need any more sugar, you're sweet enough! Okay on a serious note let's talk about some sugar facts so you know what things you should be aware of and what things you should not be afraid of. Basically, sugar gets a lot of bad rep and everyone following the diet culture is now all of a sudden highly cautious of the sugar content in food, even if they're eating fruits! Fruits are healthy! You should eat fruits and you should not be afraid of the fruit sugar or fructose that's naturally found in them. As you've just learned fruits contain beneficial vitamins and minerals!

Fruits and vegetables are rich in nutrients essential for bone health such as potassium, calcium, and magnesium. The majority of people should not be stressing over the sugar content in these foods, unless they're diabetic or have other specific reasons to do so. Fruits are low in calories, higher in fiber and higher in nutrients. They will allow you to become satiated longer help you avoid consuming excess calories. Your appetite will be controlled by the fiber and the nutrient density in the fruits so their sugar content should be the least of your worries. In other words, they will help keep you full longer with the least amount of calories.

What you should be aware of are the foods and drinks that provide you excessive amounts of sugar with no nutritional benefit whatsoever. Everything must be taken into consideration and not one specific food or item. The foods that I'm talking about are all the soft drinks, juices, candy, cakes, desserts and other sweets you eat or drink. When thinking about your daily food habits think about the amount of unnecessary sugar you have. How much sugar are you drinking in your beverages? The American Heart Association recommends that women intake about 6 teaspoons of sugar a day while men intake up to 9 teaspoons of sugar a day. That is equivalent to 25 grams (100 calories) and 37.5 grams (150 calories) of sugar, respectively.

What are some ways where you can eliminate the unnecessary sugars in your life? Once again place more emphasis on the added sugars that do not benefit you in any way besides your cravings. Do you drink juices or soda? How often? How much? Do you have way too much sugar in your coffee?

Do you drench your breakfast with syrup? Do you snack on sweets every day? What are some ways you can reduce the amount of sweets you eat and still be satisfied? Ask yourself "Can I have less?" or "What's the least amount of sweets I can have to become satisfied?"

When consuming sugars one should really avoid high fructose corn syrup. The evidence is clear on the detrimental effects it can have on your health, especially when consumed over long periods of time. It will contribute to unwanted calories that will cause you weight gain and increase your risk for health problems such as diabetes, heart disease, high blood pressure, leaky gut syndrome and so forth. Do your best to consume sugar in the most natural forms possible and shy away from the artificial sweeteners. Chronic use of artificial sweeteners has been associated with an increased risk of dementia from Alzheimer's disease.

HOW DO I LEARN PORTION CONTROL?

Now that you've learned the food breakdown essentials you have to put the information into action. You want to make sure you have your portion sizes under control if you want to be in control of your weight. Portion control is literally in your hands! In order to lose weight, you need to regulate your portion sizes of the macronutrients we discussed. Prepare to reduce the portions of foods you are currently eating throughout the day and increase your portions of high nutrient foods. Let's first talk about some ways to make your plate healthier.

You can follow these tips below:

1. Start with a smaller plate
2. Fill half your plate with vegetables
3. Choose whole grains
4. Choose lean protein
5. Choose low-fat when opting for dairy
6. Choose water as your beverage
7. Choose fresh fruit for something sweet
8. Choose a balanced meal

The Winning Wellness Method

So ideally how should a healthy plate look like? See picture below.

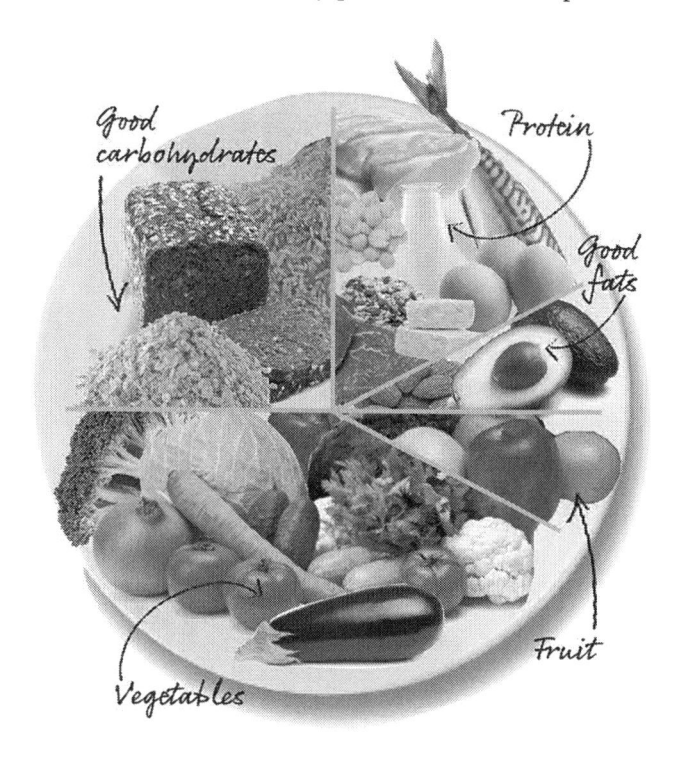

If your plate does not look somewhat similar to the picture above you can always balance it out by choosing other foods that are missing in your meal to make up for the nutrients. Balance is key and you always want to think how can you balance your meals out for it to become healthier for you. For example, if your meal does not have enough color you can always choose healthy snacks on the side to balance your plate out. Some examples may include a side of fruit with low-fat yogurt, peanut butter with sliced apples, raw veggies with hummus or some edamame.

You must balance your portions on your smaller plate with the carbs, fat and protein. Once again don't be afraid of the veggies! You may have additional greens as you wish. Remember that the higher fiber nutrient foods you have the better! You may use some tools to help you out with portioning such as measuring cups, spoons, a food scale, smaller food containers and plates. Take a look at the percentage breakdown of your plate again below.

Dr. Austin Win

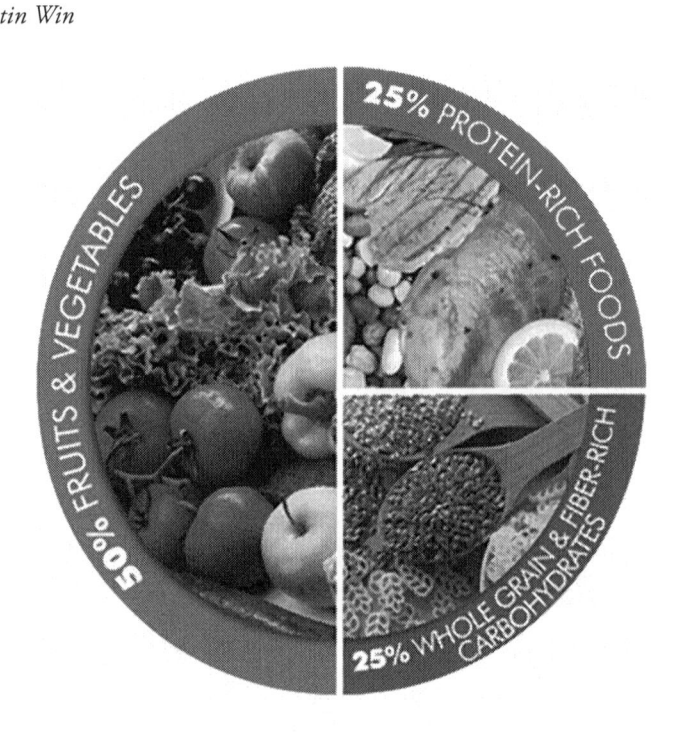

Lose the fast-processed food and disproportionate food portions! Generally speaking the typical American meal will consist of an excess of carbohydrates, sodium, fat, and sugars with little to no greens. If you analyze the typical American meal of a burger, fries and large soda you can easily see how it will pack more pounds on your body. Once more, I'm not saying to never eat these foods, but I want you to realize the impact it has on your health when you keep up with this habit over the months and years. Save these meals for the 20% of your eating patterns and know how to balance them out to make it healthier for you. Maybe you don't need to supersize everything. Maybe you can substitute some items for a healthier option. Baked sweet potato fries instead of loaded fries? Or maybe you can just eat a slider for an appetizer to fulfill your craving instead of ordering the entire burger as your entree. These are just some examples for you to think of.

Reverting back to portion control being in your hands, I will share some examples of how you can use this to your advantage. All you need is your hand! Take a look below.

1 Cup = Fist

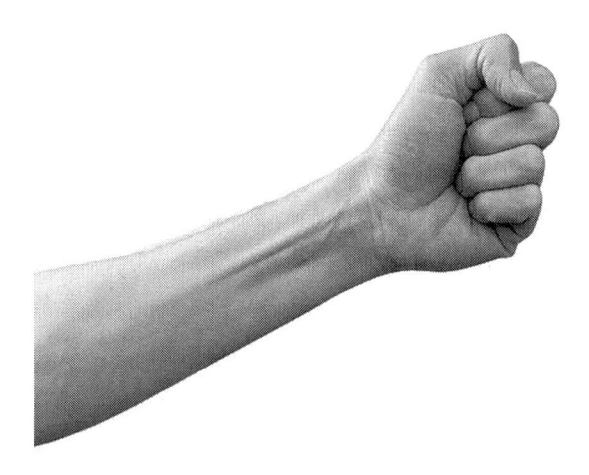

Best for:

- Cereals
- Soups
- Fresh Fruit
- Casseroles

Use your fist whenever you want to measure approximately one cup of a portion. If you know you may be eating a higher calorie food you can always use your fist to help you with the portioning. That's one trick I like to use to ensure you don't overeat unnecessary calories. Now take a look in how you can use the other parts of your hand to help you.

½ cup = Cupped Hand

Best for:
- Pasta
- Rice
- Potatoes
- Beans
- Ice cream

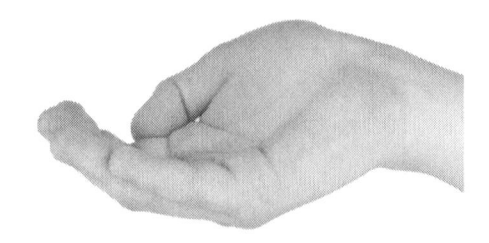

3 ounces = Palm

Best for:
- Protein
- Beef
- Poultry
- Fish
- Pork

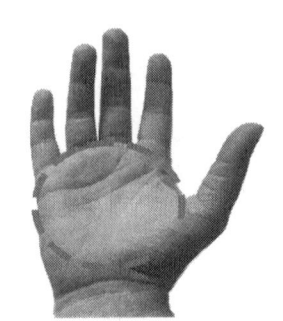

Remember your palm can equal your protein. Aim to eat lean protein the majority of the time and opt in for red meat as little as you can. If you're still hungry at the end of your meal and would like more food you can add in another serving of protein on your plate. Instead of adding more fat and carbs to the meal you can reap more benefits of the thermogenic effects of protein, while adding another side of fruits and vegetables for extra nutrients. Now let's review your thumbs.

1 Tablespoon = Thumb

Best for:
- Peanut butter
- Cream cheese
- Sour cream
- Jelly
- Salad dressing

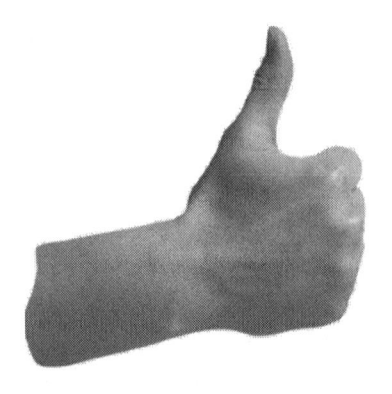

If you can control your portions you can also control your calories. You don't have to totally give up all of your favorite "bad" foods, but you should definitely be aware of the portions. You may be eating a salad and think it's healthy while pouring tons of oil or a high calorie dressing on top that will defeat the purpose of you eating a salad in the first place.

1 Teaspoon = Tip of thumb

Best for:

- Oils
- Butter
- Margarine
- Mayonnaise

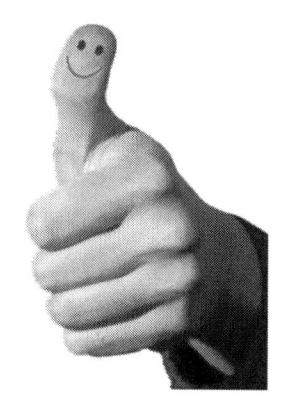

You've just learned a simple way to help you manage your portions throughout the day. Portion control must be practiced daily! It must become a good habit of yours. I firmly believe that nothing can stop you if you couple belief with action, good habits and a plan. So, in summary lose the portion distortion, choose balanced meals, practice portion control and don't forget that portion control is in your hands.

Here are 10 easy tips to help you not overeat unnecessary calories and practice portion control.

1. Plan ahead
2. Drink a big glass of water before eating
3. Eat more raw fruits and vegetables
4. Measure carefully
5. Start your meal with a soup or salad
6. Don't skip your meals
7. Slow down when eating
8. Use smaller dishware
9. Estimate your serving sizes
10. Limit Distractions

Now before you move on ask yourself what portions will you change in your meals? What portion sizes will work best for you and keep you satisfied at least 80% of the time? What measuring tools or containers do you need to support you? Think about what your portions will look like and envision them. Can you be happy and live with those portions?

FOOD TIPS TO FOLLOW

Give yourself a round of applause! We just sifted through a lot of information in the food breakdown. You have learned about carbohydrates, fats, fiber, protein, hydration, micronutrients, sugar and the importance of portion control. You also now have a better plan of how you should eat. Next you need to take all of this information and place action upon it. We will go through some more tips that will help you in achieving your goals.

Tip #1 is to make sure your goals are S.M.A.R.T. You want your goals to be specific, measurable, attainable, realistic and timely. Are your goals specific enough? Are they measurable? Can you measure your progress? Is it attainable? Is it realistic? If not, then you are setting yourself up for disaster right from the start. Lastly, is it timely? In what length of time will you reach your goals? For example, you may say "I will lose 2 pounds in one week by not drinking soda, not eating out, and adding a serving of vegetables to each meal"

Tip #2 is to not skip meals and to stick to your portion sizes that you just created. When you skip a meal, you are far more likely to overeat an excess of calories during your next meal because of your increased appetite. If you wait to eat until you are hungry then you will be more likely to binge. You don't have to dissect everything that you eat or put on your plate, but you should have the awareness of what you are putting into your body. For example, when eating try to not have piles of carbohydrates on your plate with very little fat and protein. That is not balanced. Similarly, you shouldn't have an excessive amount of fat on your plate with very little carbohydrates or protein either. Use smaller dishware to help you stick to your portions!

Tip #3 is that consistency of calories is key. It doesn't matter if you ate perfectly one day with perfect portions of macronutrients and energy dense foods or if you ate horribly one day with an excess amount of calories. What truly matters is how many days did you keep up the same habit. Did you continue to eat the same way in a week or in a month? That is what will make the big difference for you. Don't spend too much time ruminating on how you ate "bad" for one day. Decrease your calories realistically and stay consistent over time.

Tip #4 is to eat higher fiber foods to stay satisfied. When eating you can also think in terms of fiber and determine what food will give you the more of it. The more higher fiber foods you eat the more you will stay satiated and be less tempted to overeat. To make a comparison, how long will it take you to eat a Mediterranean salad versus a bowl of fried rice? It is obvious that the salad will take you a longer time to eat, which will then actually give your body the appropriate amount of time to determine if it's full or not as opposed to engulfing the fried rice and still being hungry afterwards. Think about eating beans, legumes, nuts and seeds daily!

Tip #5 is to think in terms of nutrients and ask yourself what foods will give you the most bang for your buck. Use what you have learned and make your food choices based off their nutrient value. When you are presented with food options ask yourself what food will benefit you the most. For example, when looking for a snack you can either get medium sized fries for about 365 calories with no nutritional benefit or a medium sized banana with potassium for about 100 calories. It's all about food choices and you have to make sure you consistently make good decisions.

To piggyback off thinking in terms of nutrients, Tip #6 is to start off your lunch and dinner meals with a salad. Change the sequence of eating! Raw foods will help promote weight loss and fill you up before you know it. Starting off with a salad will help slow down your eating patterns during the meal especially if you are really hungry. That will also guarantee that you get your high nutrient foods right from the beginning of eating a meal. You will not gain weight from overeating your greens!

Tip #7 is to get your five a day, meaning to eat five portions of fruits and vegetables each day. If you put tip number 6 into action and combine it with ending your meals with fruit then you would have completed about 80% of the requirement. This can easily be achieved by having fruit in your breakfast or having it as snacks during the day. You can even make a delicious frozen fruit smoothie to help get your nutrients and keep your stomach satisfied.

Tip #8 is to keep things fun! Don't keep things boring by eating the same foods every single day. I imagine there are only a limited amount of time that you can eat broccoli for every meal until you get sick and tired of it. Variety is king. Experiment with different healthy foods that you can include during the week to keep things interesting. You don't have to always use the same seasonings either. You can use fresh herbs, lemon, onions, garlic and other natural food items when creating your dishes. Combine your vegetables and mix up the flavors!

Tip #9 is to highly decrease the amount of processed foods you eat. I'm sure you may have heard to "avoid all processed foods" and although that is ideally what should be done I guarantee that the majority of people have not taken that advice to heart. Although I agree that people should avoid all processed foods, I am also a realist and know that people will continue to eat highly refined foods. I'd be very happy if you can prove me wrong! If you have implemented all of the other tips, then processed foods should be very low in your diet.

Tip #10 is to use the KISS principle, which is an acronym for "Keep it simple, stupid." Complexity is the enemy of execution! The information you have learned so far is enough for you to make better food decisions. Do not get into paralysis analysis. A healthy outside starts with a healthy inside. Use these 10 tips to your advantage and stay focused on your goals.

Weight loss does not happen overnight. It is a journey. You must think about the long game and make sure you don't do things way too fast way too soon. That is how problems occur. In terms of exercise, most people get injured and go to physical therapy because they simply did way too much way too soon. It is the weekend warriors that get themselves injured the fastest. Your body needs time to gradually change and transition, whether you're losing weight or strengthening. Your taste buds even need time to transition to the new foods!

Something I see that happens very often are people who go to the gym and start exercising intensely when they have not been to the gym in years, simply to lose weight faster. The caveat is that the same person most likely ends up getting injured and then goes to physical therapy to rehab their knee for example. They can no longer exercise due to the knee pain and ends up gaining more weight because of how inactive they've become since the injury. Keep up the pace and run your own race! The only person you should be comparing yourself to is the person you were yesterday.

A gradual pace shows that you are patient. It took a long time to put on your weight and it will take a long time to lose it. The good news is that you can give yourself a boost or kickstart with some healthy habits to ensure you start off on the right track. Would you rather have permanent results at a good steady pace or rapid results that are temporary, and that may potentially get you ill? Remember it's not a sprint, it's a marathon. Strive to continue to maintain a healthy relationship with food, which involve happiness, trust and enjoyment. Do you really want to follow a restrictive diet full of food rules and limitations when you're 60, 70 or even 80 years old? I hope not. Make small good decisions over time. Small bad decisions over time can lead to heart disease, diabetes, unnecessary joint surgeries, injections, medications and other health problems.

You have learned how to eat and what to eat to achieve permanent weight loss. You now have to figure out how you will make this all work for you. That will be the biggest challenge. Now I know I can easily tell you exactly what to eat and when to eat, but that is not what is going to help you in the long run. My goal here is to teach you how to eat and have you create a healthy life of your own. I cannot imagine anyone following an exact meal plan for the rest of their life or adhering to a specific meal plan everywhere they go. If you understand these principles that I teach you will be able to achieve food freedom and have sustained weight loss on your own terms.

CREATE YOUR OWN MEAL PLAN

Next, we will go over examples of how to create your own meal plan. I will provide some samples of a meal plan, shopping list and food recipes that you can use. Use this as a guide and work towards making your own. Think of these examples as your "training wheels" until you get in the habit of eating better so that you don't need it anymore. You wouldn't want to ride your bike with training wheels forever would you? Think of these tools as your "crutches". You eventually want to walk away from them and not ultimately depend on it. Let's first start off with the hard and complicated way to create your meal plan. This way is not necessary, but it is an option. Note: it is difficult to sustain and may cause additional stress.

Option #1: For example, you need 2,000 calories per day
Use the base formula: 50% carbs, 20% protein, 30% fat formula

Macronutrients:

1,000 calories from carbs = 250g [50% of 2,000 calories)
400 calories from protein = 100g protein [20% of 2,000 calories]
600 calories from fat = 67g fat [30% of 2,000 calories]

Then list what foods you would like to eat, break it down into 3 meals and 1-2 snacks.

Divide up the macronutrients into portion sizes, write the amount and plug into your own meal plan!

Rules to remember:

For 2,000 calories don't go over 4 carb servings per meal (Identify your carbs)
Have about 25-30 grams of protein per meal
Have about 15-20 grams of fat per meal

Serving Size

Carbs:
1/3 cup rice = 60 calories (15 g)
1 slice bread = 60 calories (15 g)
1 cup milk = 100 calories (12 g, 8g protein)

Protein:
1 oz meat = ~7g protein
1 oz beef = (7g protein, 2g fat)
1 egg = 6 g protein, 80 calories

Fat:
1 tbsp. oil/butter = 120 calories = 14g fat
1 oz nuts = 170 calories = 15g fat

Fruits & Vegetables: "**FREE**" calories [Eat Unlimited]
5-a-day = 200 calories
1 cup fruit = 50 calories
1 cup non-starchy vegetable = 30 calories

Can you imagine doing this for every single meal for every day of the week? Yes, there are easier ways to do this with the help of new applications that are out, but is this something that you truly see doing yourself? From my experience my recommendation is to not worry about it and follow the principles that I teach you in this book. If you are eating in the way that I recommend you will eventually lose weight as a result and improve your health overall. Below is an example of a 2,000-calorie plan that is significantly better than the typical American diet.

Example of a 2,000 Calorie Diet

Breakfast:
2 boiled egg
2 slices whole wheat toast
1 tbsp jam
1 cup milk
1 small banana

Morning snack:
1 orange

Lunch:
4 oz salmon
1 cup brown rice
1 cup mixed vegetables
Afternoon snack:
1 cup Greek yogurt

Dinner:
6 oz baked chicken breast
1 cup cooked pasta
1 cup pasta sauce
1 tbsp olive oil
1 tbsp parmesan cheese
1 cup cooked carrots

So, what really matters at the end of the day? First of all, you need to stay dedicated and committed towards your goals. You should be able to identify your foods and understand what you are eating. You must stay consistent with your healthy eating pattern to eat with reduced calories, eat enough protein and get your high-nutrient foods with your five-a-day. Be flexible and do not over complicate it. Progress, not perfection. Keep stepping in the right direction.

Use the weekly meal plan as an outline for you to plan your meals for the week. This will help get you started. You can use this as a framework to help guide you in the right direction as you plan your weeks out. That way you will have taken the thinking out of the process because you have planned it ahead of time. If you continue to plan your meals ahead of time you will increase your chances of success starting off. This is a great habit to have because eventually you will get to a point where you may not have to plan so much and as a result of your healthy habits you will lose weight.

WEEKLY MEAL PLAN

	Mon	Tues	Wed	Thur	Fri	Sat	Sun
Breakfast							
Mid-morning							
Lunch							
Mid-afternoon							
Dinner							
Mid-evening							

Go to www.drwinsecrets.com to see a four-week sample meal plan

Dr. Austin Win

SAMPLE CALENDAR TO KICKSTART HEALTHY HABITS

Sunday	Monday	Tuesday	Wednesday	Thursday	Friday	Saturday
	1 Clean your fridge	2 Set your intentions	2 Plan your meals	3 Add more color	4 Make a snack attack plan	5 Enjoy a latte
6 Remember to cook	7 Meatless Monday	8 Satisfy crunchy cravings	9 Make a berry good smoothie	10 Eat like a pescatarian	11 Make an awesome breakfast	12 Try new fruits
13 Try new leafy greens	14 Eat only whole grains	15 Make healthy Mexican food [TACO TUESDAY]	16 Make baked sweet potato fries	17 Add nuts in your diet	18 Balance your plate	19 Try a new salad
20 Go ahead, sample a healthy dessert	21 Add some healthy fats	22 Simplify breakfast	23 Use frozen vegetables	24 Vary your protein	25 Use fresh herbs	26 Try whole grain pasta
27 Make your favorite takeout healthy	28 Try a new healthy snack	29 Skip the fat free food	30 Use frozen fruits	31 Eat like a vegetarian		

Contact me at Austin@drwinsecrets.com

HEALTHY & EASY ANTI-INFLAMMATORY RECIPES

Refreshing Green Tea

3 Japanese Green tea bags
5-6 Fresh mint leaves
3 cups purified water

Berry Good Smoothie

1 cup unsweetened almond milk
1 cup frozen blueberries
1 tsp ground flax seeds
1 scoop protein powder
Blend and add ice as desired

Almond Butter Smoothie

¾ cup unsweetened almond milk
¼ cup spinach
2 tbsp almond butter
1 pinch of cinnamon
1 scoop protein powder

Avocado Smoothie

1 cup organic soy milk
½ cup avocado
1 scoop protein powder
½ banana

Matcha Maker

1 cup almond milk
1 cup spinach
1 frozen banana
1 scoop protein powder

2 tsp Matcha powder
½ cup ice

Supercharged Salmon Salad

Ingredients:
6 oz salmon
½ avocado
1 small tomato sliced
6 walnuts
1 tbsp Craisins (dried cranberries pomegranate infused)
1 tsp olive oil
1 lemon wedge
¼ tsp turmeric
Pinch of ground black pepper
2 cup mixed greens

Instructions:

1. Squeeze lemon wedge over salmon and apply seasonings
2. Put sauté pan on medium heat and add 1 tsp olive oil.
3. Cook salmon 3-4 minutes on each side or until a golden orange brown color
4. In a separate plate combine mixed greens, avocado, walnuts, craisins and tomato
5. Add cooked salmon on top of salad!

Would you like some more easy anti-inflammatory recipes? If so you can go to www.drwinsecrets.com and get it now. You can also receive a mini cookbook of a variety of recipes from Registered Dietitians. Included are recipes of dishes that are rich in nutrients and follow the basic principles of healthy eating. Remember you don't need to give up all of your favorite foods. You can be flexible and still lose weight, but you need to be determined.

SHOPPING LIST

Below are some ideas of healthy foods to keep in the house. Once again variety is king!

FRUITS & VEGETABLES

Buy Organic
- Apples
- Berries
- Celery
- Cherries
- Grapes
- Kale
- Nectarines
- Peaches
- Pears
- Peppers
- Potatoes
- Spinach
- Tomatoes

Fruits
- Avocado
- Banana
- Dates
- Dried Fruit
- Grapefruit
- Kiwi
- Mango
- Melons
- Orange
- Papaya
- Pineapple

Vegetables
- Artichoke
- Asparagus
- Broccoli
- Carrots
- Cauliflower
- Cucumber
- Eggplant
- Fresh Herbs (basil)
- Garlic
- Green Beans
- Mushrooms
- Onion
- Squash

The fruits and vegetables that are listed under organic are recommended because those foods have been found to be higher in pesticides. Aim to eat more of the fruits and vegetables raw than cooked because they will contain more nutrients and fiber.

CARBS

Breads
- Dave's Killer Bread
- Ezekiel Bread
- Oroweat 100% Whole Wheat
- Trader Joes' Whole Grain

Pasta
- Quinoa pasta
- Brown Rice
- Whole Wheat
- Sprouted Grain
- Vegetable Pasta

Tortillas
- Ezekiel tortillas
- Sprouted Wheat
- Organic Corn

WHOLE GRAINS

Carbs include whole grains. Try these selections to change the monotony of repetitively eating the same foods. There are more options than eating brown rice for every meal!

- Amaranth
- Barley
- Basmati rice
- Brown rice
- Farro
- Quinoa
- Millet
- Oats
- Red rice
- Wild rice

HEALTHY FATS

Oils
- Avocado
- Canola
- Coconut
- Olive
- Peanut
- Sesame

Nut Butters
- Almond Butter
- Cashew Butter
- Peanut Butter
- Sunflower Seed Butter

Nuts & Seeds
- Almonds
- Brazil Nuts
- Cashews
- Chia Seeds
- Flax Seeds
- Hemp Seeds
- Hazelnuts
- Macadamia Nuts
- Peanuts
- Pecans
- Pine nuts
- Pistachios
- Pumpkin Seeds
- Sunflower Seeds
- Walnuts

HERBS & SEASONINGS

- Basil
- Chili powder
- Cinnamon
- Complete seasoning
- Crushed red pepper
- Cumin
- Curry powder
- Dill
- Garlic
- Ginger
- Lemon Pepper
- Mint
- Mrs. Dash
- Onion powder
- Oregano
- Paprika
- Parsley
- Pepper
- Rosemary
- Thyme
- Turmeric

BEANS & LEGUMES

They are one of the most underrated foods on earth and are an excellent sources of fiber, protein, vitamins and minerals.

- Adzuki beans
- Black beans
- Black eyed peas
- Chickpeas
- Edamame
- Kidney beans
- Lentils
- Lima beans
- Pinto beans
- Split peas
- White beans

DAIRY PRODUCTS

When choosing dairy products, I recommend Greek yogurt, cottage cheese and organic cow's milk. You may also use soy, almond or coconut milk as substitutes.

PROTEIN

Remember to stay lean with protein! I recommend the following:

Grass-fed Beef
- Top sirloin
- Top round steaks
- Top loin

Fatty Fish (See Chapter 3)
- Salmon
- Herring
- Whitefish
- Cod
- Mackerel
- Sardines

Lean poultry
- Chicken breast
- Extra lean turkey

Seafood
- Shrimp
- Mussels
- Clams
- Scallop
- Squid
- Octopus
- Oysters

Others
- Beans & legumes
- Free-range eggs
- Lean pork loins
- Tempeh
- Tofu
- Venison

TAKE ACTION: PLAN FOR SUCCESS

1. Plan your meals for the week.
   - What will you eat?
   - Where will you eat?
   - When will you eat?
   - Download my cookbook if you need ideas at www.drwinsecrets.com

2. Create a shopping list. If you want a printout of the shopping list above go to www.drwinsecrets.com and download it there.

3. Go grocery shopping using your shopping list

4. Meal prep (will dive deep in Chapter 6)

5. Practice portion control with balanced meals

CHAPTER 4
NUTRITION & INJURY RECOVERY

This chapter is all about knowing how to eat when you are injured and how to use nutrition to your advantage to speed up the recovery process. We will go over common injuries that occur so you know how to incorporate weight loss during physical therapy the right way. In addition, we will go over specific foods you can add to your diet during this time and supplements you can use to help with the recovery. Before we dive into all of that, it's important to understand the different phases of healing.

There are three stages of healing and when you are injured you immediately start off with the inflammatory phase. A whole cascade of events happen during this time such as cell disruption or death when you become injured. The severity of the injury will impact the amount of cell disruption in your body. Basically during this time you have a release of pro-inflammatory chemicals and some signs are redness, swelling, heat, pain and loss of function. This phase will typically last for about 3 to 7 days, or longer.

Next is the repair phase, which starts after your injury. This is an ongoing process with inflammation, but during this time your body is laying down new tissue to the injured area and repairing damaged tissue. This is also the time period where scar tissue can form and restrict your body's range of motion. Think of these scar marks as "spider webs" that are formed during the healing process of damaged tissues to help "stabilize" the area. It's almost like a human glue-like substance that sticks to your body's muscles, tendons, ligaments and fascia. The problem is at the scar tissue is not as strong and resilient as the original tissue so this can be a time period for re injury. This phase will typically last for up to 6 to 8 weeks.

Last is the remodeling phase, which is when you are having a realignment of collagen fibers to completely restore your body's healthy function to the injured area. This is a slow and ongoing process, which may last up to one year or longer depending on the severity of the injury. During this time you want to strengthen your body to prevent re-injury and prevent any scar tissue formation. You want to maintain your flexibility in the muscles and joints and minimize the development of any chronic pain.

There are several factors that can affect your healing time, either in a positive or negative way. Some are your age, type of injury, severity of injury, medical condition, nutritional status and food intake. We will focus on the last two, which are things that you can control. My goal for this chapter is for you to understand the impact nutrition can have on your healing times.

When you are receiving rehab, you are asking the body to help heal itself on an external level. Now with nutrition you are asking your body to help heal itself on an internal level so when you add this into your regimen you have the best of both worlds. The foods you put into your body can either accelerate or delay the recovery process. When you are injured it becomes even more important to load up on nutrients to really improve healing by eating. Simply put, your goal during this time should be to certainly eliminate junk foods and add super good foods.

The severity of your injury will determine the severity of a dietary regimen you implement. If you had a more severe injury then you want to eat even more nutritious. Having a small sprain, strain or dislocation is quite different from having a bone fracture or undergoing a surgical procedure. If you did not have surgery then you will have only minor effects on your metabolism and won't need as strict of a protocol. Food is fuel for your body and it is needed for healthy repair of body tissues.

The inflammatory phase is a natural process that is needed to undergo healing. The problem occurs when the inflammatory phase last much longer than it is actually supposed to. When eating for recovery during this time you want to add anti-inflammatory foods, decrease proinflammatory foods, increase your healthy fats and add supplements as needed. You must substitute the foods that will cause your body more harm than good with jam packed high nutrient healing foods.

So, what are some foods that can cause more inflammation in your body? They are processed foods, refined carbs (white bread), fried foods (French fries), soft drinks (sweetened beverages), full-fat dairy products (ice cream), red meat, processed meat (bacon, sausage), high fructose corn syrup, alcohol, margarine, lard, shortening, vegetable oils and trans fats. If you are consuming these foods you are just adding more fire to the flame that is already there.

During the repair and remodel phase you want to focus on good high quality nutrient dense foods. You want to increase the amount of protein you eat, have a rainbow of foods, continue to avoid all the pro-inflammatory foods and add supplements to speed the healing. At the minimum you want to at least limit sugars, alcohols, fried foods, red meat and full-fat dairy products. It's not such a big concern if you are not allergic to dairy products or not lactose intolerant, but you want to make sure you limit full fat sugary foods or beverages.

Calories are very important during the healing process. Your first instinct may be to think that you need to start drastically losing weight after you had an injury to reduce your overall pain, but once again that depends on the severity of your injury. We will get to common injuries soon so you know how to solidify your nutrition plan depending on the size of the injury.

Calories are necessary to promote healing because tissue healing requires energy. Having adequate calories when you are injured will help prevent muscle breakdown, help build and repair tissue and maintain overall body balance. If you were severely injured and underwent surgery you would be doing much more harm to your body by restricting yourself of calories. You do not want to lose muscle mass in the process so this is important. You want to focus on high-quality calories versus high quantity of calories.

Again, simply substitute junk foods with whole nutritious foods. This must be a rigorous effort. If you had a basic injury such as a bruise, contusion, strain, sprain, tendonitis or dislocation then you can just tweak your food intake for the better. Your plan won't be as critical when compared to a major soft tissue injury such as a wound, fracture or post-operative procedure like a hip replacement.

Also, if you did have a major event occur you most likely would have had inpatient rehab at the hospital because those are the type of patients I saw during my work as a dietitian in acute care. More likely than not, your diet would have been regulated at the facility during that time.

In general, when you are injured I recommend to first eat for recovery, become more aware of what you're eating, become more aware of your calories and then eat for wellness and weight loss as described in the earlier chapters. The more weight you have on your body the more pressure and stress you put on your joints. Therefore, you do not want to gain weight during this time period especially if the injury has caused you to become inactive. If you had a small injury or history of on and off pain like plantar fasciitis or arthritis your calorie guidelines will not be much different from your preinjury time periods. In these cases, you want to follow the recommendations of eating during the inflammatory phase and for weight loss to reduce the stress your weight is placing on your body.

If you had severe trauma then your goal should be to first maintain your body weight and your muscle mass. You do not want to restrict yourself of the fuel needed to help repair your body's tissue. If you had a major surgery or operation then initially you will need extra calories to support the healing process. Using medium chain triglycerides or coconut oil will be an easy way to supplement the additional calories. Providing the exact calculations of nutritional requirements for musculoskeletal injuries etc. is out of the scope for this, but I can give basic generalized information for you to work with.

You first want to maintain adequate calories during the beginning phases of healing if you had a severe injury or surgery. To give a number, you'd want at least 14 kcal/lb./day. For example, if you weigh 200 lbs. you would need to consume approximately 2,800 calories a day (200 lbs. x 14 kcal). Then the goal would be to lower your calories towards the later phases of healing. This all varies depending on several factors such as your age, weight, sex, and stress factor etc. I recommend you speaking with a Registered Dietitian as they are well trained to estimate your total energy and protein needs etc.

Speaking of protein, it plays a major role in wound healing and in the recovery process. Your body needs protein and amino acids in order for it to heal. Research has shown that essential amino acid treatment can attenuate muscle atrophy and accelerate the return of mobility in older adults following a total knee arthroplasty.[13] Protein is important for collagen formation, wound remodeling and to improve overall healing. If your diet is low in protein you will have a slower healing time, more muscle breakdown, increased collagen breakdown and a prolonged inflammatory phase. Restricting food will only slow the repair process and you want to accelerate the healing, rebuild collagen and maintain as much muscle as you can.

Some basic protein guidelines during healing is to eat at least 0.5g/lb./day of protein. For example, if you weigh 200 lbs. you should consume about 100g protein a day (200 lbs. x 0.5g). For larger injuries you'd want to eat more protein, which can be up to 0.75g - 1g/lb./day. In simple terms, eat enough protein and calories throughout the day. More specifically, eat high quality protein and calories. A double cheeseburger and large side of fries do not count.

In summary, the general goals during acute healing are to first maintain adequate calories (more calories for severe injuries), add whole nutritious foods (fresh fruits, vegetables, whole grains), and remove junk foods (fried greasy foods, excess fat, sugars etc.). You want to substitute fatty red meats (hot dogs, sausages, bacon, pork cuts) for fish, eggs, or lean poultry.

Eat high-nutrient foods because they can accelerate healing of injuries. Focus on loading your body with nutrients because good nutrition can shorten the recovery time. Use food to supercharge your body! Be sure to have adequate calories and protein especially in the acute phase and more if you are severely injured. If this all seems too difficult and you feel you may need additional guidance with your specific situation, I recommend speaking with a Registered Dietitian. To find one now go to coach.drwinsecrets.com

FOODS THAT FIGHT INFLAMMATION

Research has shown that there are foods you can eat to reduce the levels of inflammation in your body. Now that you have learned the roles that nutrition can play on your body when you're injured you can see why this is important. Another alternative to taking medications and treatment is to adopt an anti-inflammatory eating pattern. Several studies have shown that a diet high in fruits and vegetables, healthy oils, whole grains, nuts, seeds, fatty fish, beans and legumes can reduce the overall inflammation in your body and lower your risk of chronic diseases.

Including anti-inflammatory foods into your meals may help with controlling pain and inflammation with conditions such as arthritis. You want to limit any foods that may trigger joint pain in your body and consume anti-inflammatory foods that can help ease your symptoms. I discourage using the term diet because more often than not it implies a short-term process, but if you examine the Mediterranean "diet" it has a whole myriad of health benefits. While there are several foods out there that are excellent to include in your "diet" during your road to good health, I will mention the top anti-inflammatory foods I recommend you start eating.

Aim to eat at least one of these foods every day. Including these anti-inflammatory foods in your "diet" will also help fight off any future inflammatory related health conditions that affect so many people worldwide. Again, this is not an end-all be-all list, but these foods have been found to give you the most bang for your buck. My goal is for you to be able to take action upon this list of top anti-inflammatory foods and start to regularly incorporate it throughout the week.

Make it a good habit to purchase these foods when going grocery shopping!

1. Blueberries
2. Nuts
3. Almonds
4. Avocados
5. Salmon
6. Cinnamon
7. Turmeric
8. Cabbage
9. Flaxseeds
10. Pomegranate
11. Garlic
12. Green tea

Blueberries are power packed with antioxidants and minerals to improve overall health. Nuts and almonds are fantastic for your heart health! They contain Vitamin E which will help reduce any plaque in your arteries. Avocados are amazingly nutritious and contain lots of potassium. They are a rich source of healthy fats. Salmon is loaded with Omega 3's and is a wonderful source of protein. It may also reduce the risk of heart disease. Cinnamon and turmeric have powerful anti-inflammatory properties as well which are a great add on to your foods. Think of them as superfood spices. Cabbage is jam packed with nutrients as it is a cruciferous vegetable. They are low in calories and will highly protect your body from cell damaging free radicals. Flaxseeds are high in fiber, antioxidants and may help prevent cancer.

They are a great addition to your smoothies and yogurt. Eating pomegranate can help protect against diseases such as Alzheimer's or cancer. They are high in Vitamin C and will totally help reduce your body's inflammation. Garlic can also reduce your blood pressure and boost your immune system. Try and start adding garlic to your foods when cooking. Choose fresh when possible! Lastly green tea has been found to have the highest level of antioxidants and contains anti-aging properties. This drink will surely reduce inflammation and may boost your metabolism too.

There you have it! My top 12 list of powerful anti-inflammatory foods! You now know exactly what to eat to help improve your body's rate of healing. I'm a big believer in letting food be your medicine. Your best medicine may be right in your refrigerator! Protect your health and immune system with these powerful inflammatory fighting foods. Adding these foods that combat inflammation is just as important as subtracting the foods that promote inflammation. Don't balance out the benefit of this list with continuing to include the wrong foods such as the sodas, french fries, white bread, pastries, alcohol, hot dogs, and sausages etc. You can download this list at www.drwinsecrets.com to print it out.

SUPPLEMENTS FOR INJURY RECOVERY

There are thousands of supplements available in the market and it may be really difficult to know which ones are actually beneficial for you. This section will specifically provide you information on what supplements you can take for injury recovery. Before we dive in, I would like to make a few things clear so that the message does not get misconstrued. I wholeheartedly believe in having food first, but most people simply do not eat a well-balanced diet. Even the most health-conscious people do not eat a perfect diet every day. Also, if you have participated in popular weight loss miracle diets in the past they all mostly translate into fewer nutrients. The fewer nutrients you have the more difficult it is to lose weight and burn body fat.

I do not support weight loss pills and will encourage the use of supplements over medications any day. The problem is that there are many claims made with different supplements and the majority of people are led to believe that "magical pills" exist to cure them of their problems. Although no one supplement alone will eliminate your specific condition, incorporating them in your life will help restore your health. Upon my own research I have provided a condensed version of supplements for you that are safe and has been proven to help speed up your recovery from an injury.

Let me provide a disclaimer: Certain nutrients are necessary during healing and can be found in foods as research has shown that not all supplements in the form of food have been proven to be beneficial. Always consult with your Physician or RD if you're on certain medications or have a certain health condition before you put yourself on a supplement plan. This is not a substitute for medical advice.

A combination of nutrients has the best potential to significantly improve the healing than a single supplement itself. When you are injured you must focus on boosting yourself up with nutrients to supercharge your body and improve your healing rate. Coenzyme Q10 (CoQ10) is an antioxidant that has been associated with weight loss and it is needed for energy production. CoQ10 can help lower inflammation, reduce your muscle injury, lower blood cholesterol levels and provide heart protective benefits.

Fish oil or Omega 3's is a wonderful anti-inflammatory supplement that is heart protective, brain protective and may help reduce cartilage breakdown. Omega 3's may reduce the enzymes that degrade cartilage so it can be beneficial for those with arthritis. If you have a medical condition and are particularly taking a blood-thinning medication I highly recommend you consult with your physician before taking supplements. Taking higher amounts of Omega 3's should only be taken under professional supervision as this nutrient has a blood-thinning effect.

Selenium is another powerful antioxidant that can help boost your immune system. It is also known as the anticancer mineral for its powerful effects. Selenium can help out with inflammatory conditions such as osteoarthritis, bursitis, tendonitis, tendinosis and low back pain. Doses of 200 micrograms daily is completely safe for long periods of time. It has been shown that selenium levels are lower in those with osteoarthritis and chronic myofascial pain.[10]

A multivitamin is a good idea to take. Consistent use of multivitamins should be taken, especially when you're at risk for nutrient deficiencies. There is no evidence of harm and the elderly can really benefit. There is a strong relationship between vitamins and chronic disease and I recommend that all adults take one multivitamin daily. A large proportion of the general population are at risk for osteoporosis, heart disease and cancer. Low intakes of vitamins in your body can contribute to this increased risk.

Glucosamine and chondroitin can help repair cartilage and improve joint pain in conditions such as arthritis. Research has shown that people have benefited from its use when experiencing joint pain. It can also help out with other conditions such as chondromalacia, tendonitis, bursitis and other traumatic injury to joints.[7] So, if you try it and you feel better then great!

Most adults, especially the elderly, are deficient in vitamin D. This can be obtained by soaking up some sun for 15 to 20 minutes a day or by consuming foods rich in Vitamin D such as fish, eggs and dairy. The other option is to take Vitamin D supplements which can help with muscle pain and improve bone health. Supplementing with Vitamin D can enhance your overall well-being and alleviate any chronic pain that may exist.[8]

I highly recommend supplementing your diet with protein, assuming that there is no contraindication in your medical history. Protein supplementation will improve your overall healing rate, enhance your recovery time after injury, and will just simply accelerate your muscle recovery. At the very least you want to maintain your muscle mass. Remember, protein is needed for muscle growth and strength.

Creatine has been shown to be one of the most studied supplements. It is naturally occurring in your body, but it can enhance rehabilitation from injuries when supplemented in your diet. Creatine has been proven to help with injury prevention, reduce the severity of an injury and accelerate post-exercise recovery.[6] Again, you must check with your physician before taking any supplements to ensure that it will be safe for you to consume. Creatine supplementation should only be avoided in certain instances such as kidney disease.

Zinc is an important mineral that is needed to stay healthy. It will improve your immune health, speed up wound healing and enhance your healing rate in cases such as bone fractures or to minimize bone density loss from immobilization. When I used to work in the hospital as an acute care dietitian, I would see patients who suffered from wounds whom greatly benefited from zinc supplementation. Not only is the evidence clear, but I saw it with my own eyes!

Vitamin E is another antioxidant that acts as a protective nutrient to help scavenge free radicals in your body. Free radicals are those bad guys that do harm to your body. Free radicals can progress your inflammation, damage your cartilage and delay healing when injured.

Supplementing with vitamin E can depress the free radical damage on your tissues in degenerative joint conditions, arthritis and chronic inflammation. It can also be used to prevent excess scar formation. Wheat germ, nuts, seeds, cereals and green leafy vegetables have higher amounts of vitamin E.

Curcumin is the active ingredient in turmeric. It has potent anti-inflammatory and antioxidant effects. It is completely safe and there are no reports of toxicity. Although I like adding turmeric to my foods with the addition of black pepper, there are supplements available that is especially beneficial for post-surgery healing. The spice is nice, but you may also purchase this in a capsule form.

Collagen is found distributed all throughout the body. Supplementing with gelatin and collagen can help with the tissue repair of your tendons, ligaments, cartilage and bone. Not only will gelatin and collagen improve your connective tissue health, it can also alleviate joint pain and specifically enhance tendon strength after injury. For example, someone with an injury to the Achilles tendon from simply doing too much too soon can benefit from this. Also, combining it with Vitamin C can enhance its healing effects.

Vitamin C is a powerful antioxidant that will protect your immune system. In regards to injuries, it can repair body tissues, improve your tendon strength and provide connective tissue protection and healing. Combining this with gelatin and collagen can be great in cases of muscle/tendon tears.[14] In terms of wound healing, combining Vitamin C and zinc can accelerate the healing time.

I will also briefly mention some "firefighting foods" as I like to call it that can aid in injury recovery. These foods have powerful nutrients and enzymes that can speed up the healing process. Dark tart cherry juice has potent anti-inflammatory effects, while papaya and pineapple have powerful enzymes for healing. Dark green leafy vegetables which include vitamin K can help out with bruises and contusions. You will have the best of both worlds when incorporating high nutrient foods with supplements.

Now when choosing supplements for injury recovery you need to ask yourself a few questions. You first need to ask yourself what is your goal? What is it that you want to achieve? What is it that you need? What injury do you have? What is the severity of the injury? From answering those questions, you can then guide yourself on what supplements will be beneficial for your individual situation.

In summary, there is no magical pill and a combination of nutrients is best. Aim for foods first and supplements second. When choosing supplements you want to start small. Don't try to incorporate everything at one time because that may not be the best solution for you. Progress, not perfection. In other words, some is better than none and you want to take only what you need. This is not an end-all be-all list, but it is my best recommendations for you to practically take action upon some of the most beneficial supplements for injury recovery.

I have created a document organizing what supplements to take to help you recover faster based off the type of injury you have. Note, if you have a minor injury and your weight is getting in the way of you recovering because of the extra pressure on your joints then you can start a plan to safely lose weight while incorporating the tips I have provided. Or if you've had chronic pain and your weight is getting in the way of you recovering as well I recommend you to start a weight loss plan and add supplements as needed. Your requirements won't be much different from your preinjury time periods, but you will have to make some positive tweaks to your eating patterns and "diet". To use this guide to help you recover from your injury in conjunction with my healthy eating recommendations go to www.drwinsecrets.com and download it now.

Once more, I recommend you speak with a Registered Dietitian to help you out with your own individualized needs and situation. A Registered Dietitian is the food expert who can best provide you with a plan including your exact nutritional requirements, especially if your medical history may be more involved. You want to ensure that there are no food-drug interactions and also guarantee a solid plan that will work best for you.

When you have a health problem you go to the doctor, not a health specialist. When you have tooth pain you go to the dentist, not a tooth specialist. When you have knee pain you go see a Physical Therapist, not a personal trainer or "rehab specialist". Likewise, when you have nutritional concerns you should go see a Registered Dietitian.

TAKE ACTION: ANSWER THESE QUESTIONS

1. What anti-inflammatory foods will I start eating more of?

2. Will I benefit from taking any supplements? If so, which ones? If you want to try a certain supplement I recommend that you talk to your physician or seek a qualified Registered Dietitian to confirm that it will be safe and effective for you.

3. Do I need help putting all of this together? If so, you can go to go to coach.drwinsecrets.com to request a qualified Registered Dietitian that can help you with your individual needs.

CHAPTER 5
OPERATION DREAM TEAM

This chapter is about helping you find support and accountability towards achieving your goals. Whenever you are facing a new challenge or taking on new goals, it makes it very difficult to go through the process alone. There will always be obstacles and difficult times that may arise and discourage you. You need a "dream team" to make sure you stay on course and not fall off track during this new journey. This dream team may consist of people or items to encourage you to continue moving forward. It's very easy to fall back into the bad habits and live on autopilot, but this chapter is designed to help you stick to your winning habits and eliminate all the self-sabotaging ones. Below are 10 tips to gaining support and accountability during your weight loss journey.

Tip #1 is to create S.M.A.R.T goals! You first want to set yourself up for success and make your goals specific, measurable, attainable, realistic and timely. Just in case you didn't do it before I am mentioning it here again. This is the first step you must take in your weight loss journey because you need to know exactly what you are striving for. With the information you have learned so far, what are your S.M.A.R.T goals now? What specific foods will you buy? What snacks will you buy? What supplements can you add?

Tip #2 is to now document your goals. You want to break down your S.M.A.R.T goals down into short term goals for the day and the week. You want to write them down and make yourself accountable for what you said you were going to achieve. Review them often to see if you were successful or unsuccessful and strategize on what needs to be improved.

The Winning Wellness Method

One easy way to do this is to carry a small notebook with you at all times so that your goals can stay in the forefront of your mind. At the end of the night you can take a look to see if you have accomplished your daily goal.

Tip #3 is to write it on the calendar. Does your calendar reflect your priorities? Having your goals written down on the calendar will give you a good picture of what you will have to do in order to achieve your goals. Your calendar will be your road map and will help you stay accountable. This calendar can be placed somewhere easily visible like on your refrigerator so that you are sure to see it every day. You can even cross off your goals on the calendar so you can motivate yourself each day and week every time you accomplish them.

Tip #4 is to journal daily. Journaling will help support you and increase the likelihood of you achieving your goals. You want to write down your thoughts, your successes, challenges and obstacles. This will help you find clarity and peace within your mind on what is actually happening during this journey. Sometimes it can be too easy to be caught up in the forest that you can't see past the trees. In other words, journaling will help you oversee the mountain you are climbing. The simple act of keeping a food diary can help you lose weight. Did you know that you can lose 38 lbs. in 3 years by simply eating 120 calories less a day? If you journaled that your goal was to only eat 120 calories less a day or to eat one less chocolate a day you can lose 38 lbs. in 3 years by that one simple change. Now imagine the possibilities if you made even bigger changes!

Tip #5 is to ask a friend. It is difficult to go through this process alone and there is nothing wrong and asking for help and support. Go ahead and ask your friend, family member or your significant other to go on this winning weight loss journey with you and be your accountability partner. When choosing an accountability partner, you want to make sure that the person you pick will be trustworthy, be able to challenge you and actually keep you accountable.

You and your accountability partner can then schedule meetups and have planned meals together instead of eating out sporadically. At the bare minimum I recommend you have weekly talks with your accountability partner and share your S.M.A.R.T goals with them!

Without a support system you will have to be extremely disciplined and relentless towards achieving your goals. It is much easier if you have someone helping you, coaching you or just going on the journey with you. When you do find your accountability partner you must not forget that you still have to take responsibility for yourself. You do not want to put any blame on anyone else but yourself. You are ultimately accountable for your own actions. Please take personal responsibility and ownership of your own decisions. Revisit your WHY frequently with your accountability partner and keep the motivation going!

Tip #6 is to find or join a community. Find like-minded people in your similar situation and join them. There is power in numbers! Announce your goals to the community. Participate in some friendly challenges to motivate you. One example is a healthy eating group where everyone is sharing their journey to new health. It's exciting and motivating to see that there are others just like you going through the same adventure. That is why I created a private group online for everyone who has gone through my Winning Wellness Method course. Positive energy is contagious and the impact in can have on you is incredibly powerful!

Tip #7 is to create your own community. Can't find a community to join? No problem. You can create one of your own. Who else do you know that can benefit from losing some extra weight and fat off their belly? Take the lead and have them come join you. Have them read this book so that they too can benefit and understand everything you're learning. You can create a nice little community in your town for people to join in on the winning wellness journey. Make it fun! I must warn you though. You must be aware of the negative thoughts and conversations in your community. You are the average of the five people you spend the most time with. Make sure you aren't being anchored down with negative energy and people who do not have the same goals as you. You want the power of influence to work for you and not against you.

Tip #8 is to create the right environment. Creating the right environment is the key to success. How can you eat "clean" when you have a "dirty" refrigerator? Steer yourself away from all temptation. Clear out junk foods and add in whole nutritious foods in your house. Your dream team isn't only composed of your support system and or accountability partner. It also includes your environment. You need certain things in your environment to remind you to stay on track and not fall off course. You need to include certain cues in your environment to trigger you to take a positive action and then get rewarded on it from successfully completing the action.

Some examples of cues that you can implement are post-it notes where you can write positive affirmations and quotes on it to help you meet your goals. These post it notes can be placed in highly visible areas such as your door, desk, refrigerator, car or computer. This can be something as simple as writing "I will have my five servings of fruits and vegetables today" on a post-it note and sticking it on your front door so that you are sure to see it before you walk out of the house. If you successfully accomplish your goals for the week, or whatever time frame you create, you can have a reward attached to it that you really look forward to. Preferably it will not be a food reward, but it will be something that is really meaningful to you and that you crave. For example, a reward for meeting your goals can be to get a nice massage or go to the spa for the day. Whatever it is that you truly desire, go ahead and make it a reward for when achieving your goals. This can be weekly, biweekly or monthly rewards. The decision is up to you. Remember you have to celebrate the small wins!

Going back to creating the right environment, some things I highly recommend you do is purchase a hydro flask, lunch box, portioned containers, meal prep items, smaller dishware, blender, measuring tools (spoons, cups etc.), and a food scale. These are items I recommend you purchasing to put into your environment at the bare minimum. These will all help support you on your journey, help you save time and ultimately save you calories. Having a hydro flask in sight will bring more awareness to yourself to make sure you stay hydrated throughout the day. Having a lunch box in sight will encourage you to prepare and pack your meals during the week. Having portion containers and smaller dishware will ensure that you don't go over your portions. A food scale is great to have in the beginning to make sure you know what your portions are for certain foods. Having a blender in sight will also encourage you to create healthy smoothies. Say for instance one morning you "didn't have time" to make breakfast and considered skipping a meal. Well if you have a blender in sight you can at least prepare a healthy shake to go in less than one minute! All these items will be your heroes in the kitchen.

Tip #9 is to get exercise gear. You are more likely to exercise if you have exercise clothes and shoes in the first place. You can buy a gym bag and fill it with your exercise gear. Having this ready in sight will help support you even on the days when you don't feel like exercising. You can even purchase some exercise equipment such as dumbbells to encourage you to exercise at home. Just make sure you don't store your exercise gear in a closet where it can be easily forgotten and get lost in a land far far away. You want to put your exercise gear in places that you are most likely to see it, such as in your car so that you can be ready to exercise each day with no excuses.

Tip #10 is to invest in a Registered Dietitian. I cannot emphasize this enough because they are the food experts that can best help and support you on your weight loss journey, especially if you have a medical condition. Investing in a Registered Dietitian to help coach you can best keep you accountable to eat better and lose weight without the guilt of eating "bad" foods. You want to always look out for those who have your best interest at heart and I assure you that all my Registered Dietitians do. If you spend time with people who give out ridiculous advice you will be sure to do ridiculous things for your health and that is what I'm hoping you avoid.

Having a Registered Dietitian on your dream team is an invaluable asset. They will not take the cookie cutter approach towards your health. It may be the greatest investment you can ever make when going on this journey to lose weight and avoiding the diet mentality. If you haven't visited yet, go to coach.drwinsecrets.com to find a Registered Dietitian who can help you with your specific needs.

TAKE ACTION: GET READY FOR SOME MORE WINS

Answer the following questions before you move onto the next chapter. To see the true value in this you must take action. Knowledge alone is not power, execution is!

Who will be my accountability partner? Why?

What will be my cues and triggers? (Example: Leaving fruit on dining table)

1.
2.

3.
4.
5.
6.
7.
8.
9.
10.

What items do I need to help me be successful in reaching my goals? (Example: lunchbox, containers, measuring utensils?)

1.
2.
3.
4.
5.
6.
7.
8.
9.
10.

CHAPTER 6
KITCHEN FRIENDLY COOKING

Food and cooking have always been a passion of mine. It's actually one of the big reasons on how I got started into the nutrition and dietetics profession. When I first started cooking I had no idea how to make healthy meals. As a matter of fact, I didn't know how to cook much food in general, but I was determined to learn. I wasn't given any instruction or guidance and so I found resources to help me on my journey to healthy cooking. I started working in restaurants and watching the Food Network as if it were a TV series marathon. As I started learning what to eat and how to eat to become healthy, I also became committed on learning how to cook healthy as well.

This path led me to become a sushi chef for over a decade. Throughout college I found myself expressing my creative and artistic side through sushi, which is definitely an art form in itself. Cooking was an enjoyable activity to me and I really didn't consider it a chore. I found joy through creating different dishes and used cooking as a form of an "escape" or a stress relieving activity. It was certainly a challenge in the beginning to cook new dishes and consistently prepare my meals. I found that the real challenge was in the kitchen and not in the gym!

Some of you may be thinking right now, "Well that's good for you Dr. Win, but what if I don't like cooking?". If you're asking that question in your head then you must be prepared to either spend more money to have your meals prepared for you, spend more money to buy foods at healthy restaurants, or start learning to cook in a way that is both enjoyable and sustainable for you. Or hopefully you have a close friend or loved one who can do all of this for you. I don't expect everyone to have a love or passion for cooking like I did, but my point is that you don't have to. You don't need to be a professional chef or cook to create simple healthy dishes at home. It may seem like a daunting task to do, especially if you don't like cooking or think that you aren't good at it, but I'm telling you that your transformation will happen in the kitchen. Start off with simple and easy recipes that you can make. Every dish does not need to be a gourmet meal!

YOU DON'T HAVE TO BE A 5-STAR CHEF TO COOK

When I started cooking I did follow some recipes, but I was never great at it. I realized that most recipes do not have to be followed exactly and can actually be modified to your personal preferences. When I say this, I mean in terms of flavor, not the actual temperature of cooking a food. For the most part a recipe provides you with the steps to perfectly create the dish, but it does not mean that you can't add or subtract things from it. I remember I would glance at recipes and "wing it" when it came to making certain meals. If I messed up and it was a complete fail then I learned from it. It gave me the freedom to create meals I liked and challenged me to experiment in the kitchen. You too can use recipes to get you started cooking and when you feel like you have the hang of it you will no longer need to depend on them, unless you're making something for the very first time. If you consistently cook simple and easy dishes all you would have to do is mix up your seasonings to change the flavors of your meals.

You don't want to feel like you're eating the same exact thing every single day. Cooking may feel difficult to do in the beginning, but I promise you that if you constantly work to get better at it the easier it will become. If you like challenges I challenge you to start making a habit of creating more meals at home. It will save you more calories, more money and your health in the long run because you know exactly what you put into your foods. During college I ended up loving the art of cooking so much that I opened a small restaurant with my family in Miami, FL called Jasmine Sushi & Thai Cuisine. I included some of the best tasty healthy dishes you could ever eat! You never know how much you may enjoy cooking too so I challenge you to start experimenting more in the kitchen.

LET'S GET COOKIN'

Now let's start talking about some healthy ways of cooking and how you can best set yourself up for success in the kitchen. There are basic cooking techniques that you can incorporate to make healthy meals without buying expensive equipment. These healthy cooking techniques allow you to keep more of the nutrients in foods without adding excess fat to it.

These cooking methods include baking, boiling, braising, broiling, grilling, roasting, sautéing, steaming and stir-frying. Although these are all of your options, it does not mean that you have to include every single method when you cook during the week.

Baking generally doesn't require you to add large amounts of fat, unless you're making desserts. You can use baking to help you cook almost anything. The best part of it is that the food will be cooking in the oven and you don't have to be right over it the whole time. You could be doing other tasks such as washing dishes while your food is baking. I like baking foods because it is easy and convenient. You don't have to physically be cooking the meal and stay right over the stove top as compared to stir-frying. You're also able to cook large amounts of food when you bake it in the oven. That may be a good option for preparing your meals for the week.

When you choose to boil foods, you don't need to add fat in there either. It is a very simple method of cooking that you can use for eggs, vegetables, meat, soups, stews, seafood, rice, potatoes and noodles. It will help you preserve most of the nutrients in the food when compared to other methods of cooking such as frying. Mildly blanching of your vegetables will also help retain more fiber and nutrients. Some foods may not be able to be eaten raw so in those cases boiling them would be a good choice.

Braising is a combined cooking method that consists of dry and wet heat. It involves first searing or browning the food at a high temperature in a pan, and then it is finished in a covered with small amounts of liquid. This method of cooking involves a little more work, but it helps tenderize the ingredients while maintaining the natural flavors of the food. Braising is a good option for tougher cuts of meat, but a bad option if you don't have much time to cook. Besides fish and vegetables, it may take several hours to cook most braised dishes.

Broiling and grilling are both good ways to cook food while allowing excess fat to drip away. You can either grill food outdoors or indoors. When deciding where you should grill you should factor in the amount of food you have and the amount of time you have to cook. If you don't have that much time to cook and only have small portions of food to make, then indoor grilling may be best with a nice portable electric grill. Broiling uses direct heat to cook and can be done by placing foods on a broiler rack under an electric coil. It involves the heat source over the food as opposed to under it and requires the food to be turned during the cooking process to cook one side at a time.

Roasting is almost like baking, but the difference is that roasting usually involves higher temperatures with foods that have a solid structure. It may be one of the easiest cooking techniques. For example, you would roast a whole chicken in an uncovered roasting pan in the oven. The dry hot air will cook it evenly on all sides. You can also roast vegetables such as broccoli, squash, zucchini, bell peppers and potatoes. This is another hands-free cooking method that will allow you to do other things like spend time with your family while the oven is doing the cooking for you.

Sautéing involves adding some fat over high heat in a pan to quickly cook food. I recommend adding minimal amounts of fat such as olive oil when sautéing foods. Don't forget to portion the oils out! This is a basic cooking method that is often used in the kitchen. You may also use a good quality nonstick pan to minimize the use of extra fats in your cooking. Whether it's meat or vegetables, it's important that the foods you sauté are more naturally tender because the time spent in the pan is somewhat brief. I love sautéing garlic and onions with most meals of the meals I make, both for their wonderful taste and healing properties.

Steaming is a healthy way of cooking that works by continuously boiling water while the steam itself will cook the food above. This cooking method is mostly used to cook vegetables in a steamer or in a colander above boiling water. The food is in direct contact with the steam and kept separately from the water, giving it a moist texture to the food when it is complete.

Stir-frying involves cooking foods in high heat in a lightly oiled pan while continuously stirring the foods. This method of cooking involves you to be directly over the stove top to make sure you do not burn your food.

The majority of Chinese restaurants include massive amounts of oil when stir-frying and therefore is not healthy. You can make plenty of healthy dishes at home when you portion out the amount of oil that you include in your foods. One example is a quick and easy combination of chicken stir-fry. There are many quick and healthy easy recipes available.

HOW DO YOU MEAL PREP ON A BUSY SCHEDULE?

Now that you know what the healthy methods of cooking are, you need to create an organized system for yourself. You need to find out what days you will do the majority of your shopping and cooking. Throughout my experiences, having designated days of bulk shopping and cooking is a very effective strategy. This is what also occurs in restaurants. The restaurant will have major delivery days where large amounts of food come in to be stored and the cooks will also have a day where the majority of food preparation occurs. Afterwards, shopping and food preparation is done during the week as needed.

Meal preparation is key. I like to choose Sunday as the day where I prepare the bulk of my meals. I do my best to prepare as much food as I can for the week so that I don't need to spend large amounts of time cooking each day.

There are foods that I prepare in large amounts and others that I cook right before I eat. This all depends on your certain situation and preference. If you have the time to cook and want to eat your foods fresher I recommend cooking right before you eat your meal. If you don't have much time during the week and you don't care to reheat your foods, then I recommend to batch cook your food ahead of time.

Before you cook you need to know what you are going to eat. This involves you making your own shopping list and choosing a day to do most of your grocery shopping. I tend to do my bulk shopping the same day as I do my bulk cooking. You can choose how you would like to arrange this as it does not have to be the same day. It is just my preference to make one trip and get most of my shopping and cooking out of the way. I usually buy about 1-2 weeks' worth of food and buy smaller items during the week as needed, such as the condiments, spices, herbs, milk, and certain fruits and vegetables. You want to make sure you purchase what you can finish. I only buy foods that I know will be completed in my household. For example, if something is on sale and the amount of food is too much for me to eat before it expires I will not buy it. On the other hand, if it is an item that I can store or freeze to use at a later date I will purchase it.

Here are some more examples of foods that I will buy when bulk shopping: grains, canned items, bread, eggs, nuts, meat, seafood, yogurt, healthy snacks, fresh or frozen fruits and vegetables. You must first decide what you want to eat and then create a list of items to purchase that you know you can finish in a specified period of time. If you finish a food earlier than expected or run out of a particular item during the week you can go to a small grocery store instead of going to a wholesale for bulk shopping. For example, when I go to a wholesale like Costco or BJ's I make sure that I can finish the foods before they go bad in order to reduce waste. If I don't believe I can eat a dozen apples in a week I will not buy those apples in bulk.

You want to buy those type of perishable items in smaller amounts, otherwise you'll have tons of expired food in your house. To save yourself some more time in the kitchen with meal preparation, you will want to portion out some foods such as your fish and meats. I like to buy my meats and fish in bulk. I make sure to portion them out correctly and place the extra amounts of fish or meat in the freezer to use at a later time. I will leave out the meat I know I can finish during the week in the refrigerator and take out the portioned meats from the freezer when I plan to eat them. That way I have completed my meat preparation when portioning them out and saved myself another trip to the grocery store. Not to mention the time I also saved myself from washing more dishes!

You have to think of ways you can maximize your time in the kitchen. Although this is not the ultimate guide to cooking, I will provide you with simple tips and advice that has worked out for me and my clients. If you know what meals you will have for the week, then you know what food items to prepare for the week. An example of some meal preparation is to cut your onions in larger amounts ahead of time. That way you can save the extra onions you prepared for cooking during the week instead of preparing them right before the meal each and every day. This can also be done with other vegetables as well such as your bell peppers, broccoli, carrots, celery etc.

It's ultimately up to you to decide how you want to batch cook. You can do this completely 100% before the week starts, or even do it 75%, 50% or 25%. The question is how much time do you want to spend cooking during the week? Do you want your foods made really fresh? Do you mind reheating your foods?

If you do not mind reheating your foods then you can do the majority of the cooking in one day. You can even prepare your cooked vegetables, protein and grains ahead of time in portioned containers. That way all you would have to do is reheat your meals when it came time to eat. Not much time would have to be spent during the week to cook because you would have already 100% completed it. If you don't mind your foods being semi fresh you can always batch cook your grains and have the protein and vegetables cooked last "on the spot". That way those foods would be freshly made right before you eat and the grains can just be reheated for the week. Meal preparation can be done in many ways. The way I do it may not work for you and vice versa. Everyone's lives are different so I can only share certain principles that you can adopt in your own life. You need to find a way that is both effective and sustainable for you.

Start off by choosing a few items that you want to eat for the week. Make those meals beforehand and have it ready for you to eat so that you don't have to cook every single day. Afterwards you can repeat the process so you have additional meals to eat for the next few days. Like I said, there are many ways to do this. Think about how you can save time in the kitchen. If you are going to use similar ingredients over and over during the week, it only makes sense to prepare them all at one time. A food processor can help you save time with slicing, grinding and preparing foods than manually doing it with a knife. An indoor grill can also help you save time when cooking smaller food items such as grilled salmon, vegetables, or lean turkey burgers.

Properly grocery shopping is another crucial part to your success. Please go to the end of Chapter 3 for a reminder of a healthy eating shopping list. You will be responsible for the kinds of foods that you bring into your house. That is why it's important to create a list beforehand so that you can stick to it when you go shopping and not be persuaded by all of the things that you see. I know it can be very tempting to rationalize why you need a certain food, even though you know you should not buy it. Remove the temptation right from the beginning. Out of sight out of mind.

If it's not on the grocery list it should not be going in your cart! You also want to avoid going to the grocery store hungry because you most likely will be very tempted to buy more than you need. Have a plan in mind so that you are not randomly buying everything that is presented to you. If you set your kitchen up for success you are giving yourself a much better chance of achieving your goals because of all the nutritious foods you have purchased.

Another tip when going grocery shopping is to set a time limit for yourself. If you budget the amount of time you will spend at the grocery store you will also save yourself extra time by not buying the unnecessary items that were not on your grocery list. You may be tempted to buy the deals that are going on, but you have to ask yourself if you can finish those foods before they expire and if those foods will even improve your health. Aim to buy more fresh fruits and vegetables and double-check to make sure they are in good shape, literally. Feel free to explore through the produce section and try out a new fruit or vegetable to keep things interesting!

Buying produce that are in season are both fresh and delicious! To download my list of fruits and vegetables to purchase based on the season go to www.drwinsecrets.com. When going grocery shopping it is important to understand the basics in regards to nutrition labels so that you can make better informed food choices for your health. I will briefly give an overview on nutrition labels so that you can make quick, effective and easier decisions when grocery shopping.

BE SAVVY AT THE SUPERMARKET

Let's first start with the serving size. This is the first place you should look at when checking out a food label. The size of the serving and the amount of servings in the food package will influence how many calories there are. This is typically the area that most people overlook and will become deceived when buying the food. For example, if you ate the entire package above you may initially think that you consumed only 90 calories, when in fact it will be 90 calories x 4 servings. Don't get fooled! Pay attention to the serving size and servings per container.

Next you should check your calorie section of the label. Remember that your portions or serving sizes will determine how many calories you actually intake. You can help manage your weight and make better decisions when you check how many calories the food provides. Some general guidelines when looking at the calories is that 50 calories is low, 100 calories is moderate, and > 400 calories is high. Purchase items that are in the low to moderate end, especially with snacks. Eating too many sneaky calories in your day can cause you to gain more weight.

Thirdly, you want to look at the nutrient section and limit the total fat (saturated fat, trans fat), cholesterol and sodium. As part of a balanced diet you want to keep those nutrients as low as possible because they will do more harm to your health than good. You then want to look below and get enough of the nutrients that most Americans do not get, which are the fiber, vitamins and minerals. For example, getting enough calcium in your diet can reduce your chances of any bone fractures from osteoporosis. You can use this section to both limit the bad nutrients and increase the good nutrients in your daily life.

Afterwards you can look at the footnote section at the bottom of the food label, which will predominantly be the same. It is a required statement on all food labels, which will basically show the recommended dietary advice and daily values for each of the nutrients based off a 2,000 or 2,500 calorie diet. You will see the recommended goal, daily value and percentage daily value. For example, in the footnote section under the column of 2,000 calories the recommended goal is for you to consume less than 65g fat, 20g saturated fat, 300 mg cholesterol, and 2,400 mg sodium. It is also recommended that you eat at least 25g fiber if you're on a 2,000-calorie diet. This will serve as a good reminder to see how the food you're choosing compares to what is generally recommended.

Lastly, you want to look at the % daily value, which tells you the daily value recommendations of nutrients on a 2,000-calorie diet. You can use this as a frame of reference to determine if a food is high or low in a certain nutrient. You can also use the % daily value to help compare different products or brands when choosing similar food items. Use this section to help you balance yourself when eating one of your favorite foods that may be higher in fat. You can then balance it out with items that are lower in fat in the day to make sure you don't go over your % daily value.

A quick and easy tip is to remember that 5% or less is low and 20% or more is high. If you are looking to increase your intake of calcium to help keep strong bones you will want to achieve 100% daily value of calcium. In the example of the food label above, calcium is at 2% of your daily value and therefore is very low in calcium! You would need 50 servings of this food to achieve 100% of your calcium intake for the day (2% x 50 = 100%).

This is a basic guide to get you started, but go to www.drwinsecrets.com to download my food labels document. You can print it out as a guide and bring it with you when you go shopping!

In chapter 5 we spoke about the importance of creating the right environment. Your kitchen is a big part of your environment. After all, how can you expect to eat "clean" if you have a "dirty" kitchen or refrigerator? I have a kitchen makeover list to give you some ideas to help you set up your kitchen so that you can have success. It will include items to store in your pantry, list of foods to store in the refrigerator and some foods that are okay to store on your counter. Having a winning kitchen will help improve your shopping, storing, cooking and eating habits. You're setting your environment up for success!

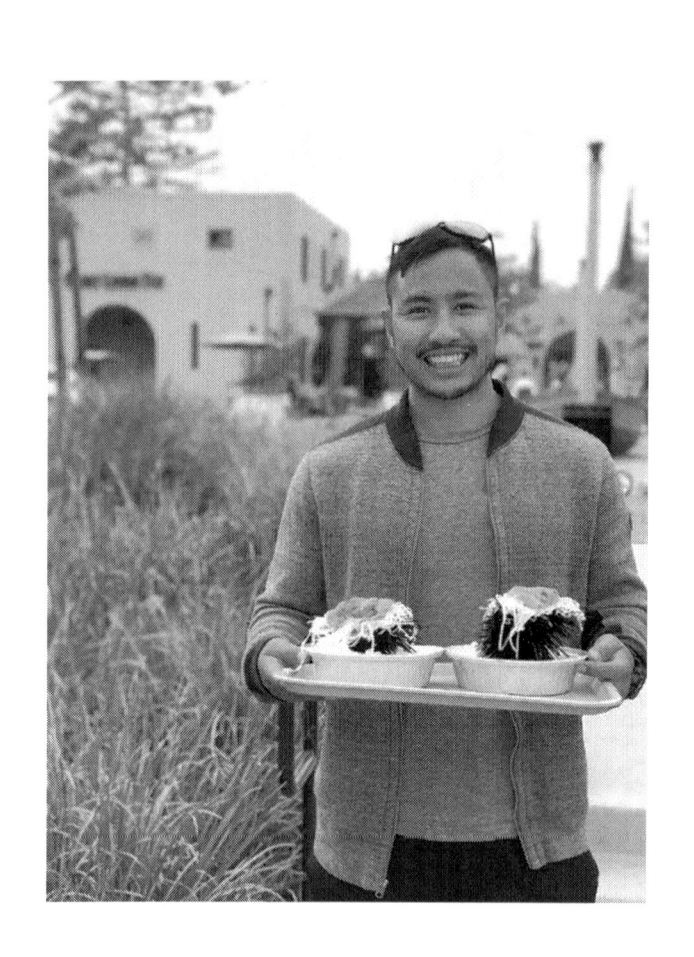

Your Kitchen Makeover Checklist

Do You have:

1. Pictures of your goals on the refrigerator?
2. Visible grocery list?
3. Storage system?
4. Healthy recipes or easy-to-read cookbook?
5. Measuring tools (cups, spoons, scale)?
6. Distractions (TV in eating area)?
7. Clean kitchen table (Free of clutter)?
8. Spice rack and spices?
9. Water Filter?
10. Fresh fruits or healthy snacks on counter?

<u>List of foods to store in your pantry</u>

Increase the shelf life of these foods by keeping them away from light

- Garlic
- Onions
- Potatoes
- Shallots
- Sweet potatoes
- Hard winter squashes

<u>Key tips</u>

- Make a master plan to buy, defrost and cook all foods
- Wash hands before and after handling foods
- Refrigerate leftovers within two hours of preparation

<u>List of foods to store on your counter & can then go into the refrigerator if necessary</u>

- Avocados
- Apricots

- Bananas
- Kiwi
- Mangos
- Nectarines
- Papaya
- Peaches
- Pears
- Pineapple
- Plums
- Tomatoes

List of foods to store in the refrigerator

- Apples, artichokes, asparagus
- Beets, berries
- Cabbage, carrots, cauliflower, celery, cherries, citrus fruits, corn, cucumbers
- Eggplant
- Fresh herbs
- Grapes, green onions, greens
- Leeks, lettuces
- Mushrooms
- Peppers
- Radishes
- Spinach, summer squash
- Turnips
- Zucchini

This is a great list for you to have so that you can organize the foods in your kitchen. If you want to print it out you can go to www.drwinsecrets.com and download it now.

Take a moment to think of how your kitchen looks like. Is there anything that can be improved? Is your kitchen working for you or against you? How can you make your kitchen work for you?

The Winning Wellness Method

Below are some ideas and action steps you can take to improve your kitchen!

FIXIN' THE KITCHEN

1. Clean and organize your pantry and cupboards throwing old expired stuff
2. Move commonly used items to the front
3. Group together the canned items (fruits, veggies, tomato products, canned meats)
4. Clean and organize the refrigerator and freezer
5. Designate a specific shelf, drawer and area for your frequently used items
6. Make a special place for your fruits and vegetables
7. Don't pack the refrigerator too tight!
8. Defrost meat in the lower shelf of the refrigerator.
9. Make sure all of your appliances are accessible, clean and in working order
10. Have a storage system for leftovers
11. Label your shelves so you know exactly where your ingredients are
12. Create a leftover storage system (freezer bags, storage containers, label and date)
13. Untangle the utensil drawer (spatulas, knives, measuring spoons, cups etc.)
14. Place cookbooks in plain view and not stuffed
15. Have two cutting boards (one for meat and one for produce)

Congratulations! You now have a new and improved kitchen. Use the steps above to help you create a kitchen success system. Now that you have the tools and kitchen environment setup you are far more likely to sustain your healthy eating habits. You don't have to implement each step listed. Just select the biggest things that will help you out the most and do them. Now let's go through some simple and easy healthy recipes you can make at home. This is by no means an extensive recipe book, but I want to give you some examples of healthy recipes that don't involve a lot of time or effort to make. You can get a free copy at www.drwinsecrets.com.

EASY HEALTHY RECIPES

Pomegranate-Powered Smoothie

1 cup pomegranate juice
½ cup almond milk
½ cup frozen blueberries
½ cup frozen strawberries
1 scoop protein powder
1 tablespoon chia seeds
<u>Instructions</u>: Blend all the ingredients in a blender until a smooth consistency

Holy Guacamole

2 peeled and pitted ripe avocados
½ cup finely chopped red onion
½ cup finely chopped tomato
½ cup minced cilantro
2 tablespoons fresh lime juice
¼ teaspoon freshly ground black pepper & sea salt to taste
<u>Instructions</u>: Mash the avocados in a bowl and then stir in the remaining ingredients.

Asian Pear Salad

6 cups mixed greens & 1 cup arugula
2 Asian pears, peeled, cored and sliced
¼ cup dried cranberries or Craisins
¾ cup chopped walnuts
2 tablespoons rice vinegar
2 teaspoons olive oil
1 lemon
Sea salt & freshly ground black pepper to taste
<u>Instructions</u>: Combine all ingredients in the bowl and mix well.

Spicy Sautéed Chicken

12 oz. chicken breast cut into small strips
1 tablespoon olive oil
1 cup chopped tomatoes
1/2 cup chopped green bell pepper
½ cup chopped red bell pepper
1/2 cup chopped onion
1 tablespoon minced garlic
2 tablespoons complete seasoning
¼ teaspoon crushed red pepper

Instructions:

1. Heat sauté pan on medium heat. Add oil, garlic, onions, peppers & cook for 3 min
2. Add chicken and cook for 5 minutes.
3. Add tomatoes and seasonings. Bring to a slight boil over high heat.
4. Reduce heat to simmer on low heat, covered for 10 minutes.

Chicken and Vegetable Stir Fry

2 tablespoons coconut oil
1 tablespoon minced garlic
½ cup chopped onions
2 cups chopped mixed vegetables
12 oz. chicken breast cut into small strips
2 tablespoons reduced sodium soy sauce
½ teaspoon ground black pepper
1 tablespoon complete seasoning
Mixed vegetable ideas:
Carrots and celery
or
Broccoli, carrots and red pepper

Instructions:

1. Heat oil on medium heat in a pan to sauté. Add onions and garlic. Stir up to 1 min.
2. Add chicken strips and continually stir for 6 minutes. Turn heat to medium-high.
3. Add mixed vegetables and stir for 2 minutes or until desired softness
4. Add reduced sodium soy sauce, complete seasoning, ground black pepper and mix.

TAKE ACTION: GET YOUR COOKING APRON ON

1. Fix the kitchen. Go through the kitchen makeover list and see what things can be tweaked in your home to set your environment up for success.

2. Select your cooking methods. Decide what cooking methods you want to try that will be both healthy and easy for you to do.

3. Master your meal preparation. Create a schedule and plan that you can consistently perform each week. See what items you can purchase that will make your meal prep life easier.

4. Get cooking! Now for the fun part. You get to cook your own food and play in the kitchen. Try out some of the easy healthy recipes above! Take pictures of your master creation and post them up on Instagram. Just make sure to tag me @draustinwin and use the #winningwellness so that I know you took action.

5. Need a cookbook? If you haven't downloaded it yet, I have created a mini cookbook with other Registered Dietitians including some easy, healthy and tasty recipes you can create at home. You can get it now at www.drwinsecrets.com and use it to stir up some ideas!

CHAPTER 7
THE WINNING SECRETS

What's the secret to weight loss? That's the big question that everyone wants to know. Although I would like to tell you that there are big and mysterious secrets to losing weight, the truth is that there really isn't. Nutrition plays a major role in your ability to lose weight, but that isn't the only factor. Please notice that I continue to use the term "nutrition" and not "diet" because the word diet implies that it is temporary.

The "secret" is that you must take everything into consideration to truly be successful in losing weight and achieving an overall healthy life. That includes nutrition, exercise, stress management, mental wellness and sleep. These are the winning secrets! If you're consistently doing extremely well and rating very highly in each of these areas then I have no doubt that you will lose weight. The hard part is to actually start building the momentum, but once you do it can turn into a habit that will serve you for the rest of your life. According to research, building a habit takes somewhere between 21-66 days so I recommend to start with the ONE thing that will make the biggest difference for you.[2]

Nutrition, exercise, stress management and sleep are the categories that you must be successful in to truly win in your wellness and have a healthy weight! We will discuss several tips and tricks you can take action on right away to improve yourself in these areas. You must take everything into consideration for your health to be successful in the long term. One of my favorite quotes is that "If you don't make time for wellness, your body will sure make time for illness".

THE LOST ART OF POSITUDE

There are six things that you must incorporate to win in your wellness. They are positivity, planning, preparation, consistency, dedication and commitment. Let's start with the 3 P's, positivity, planning and preparation. As human beings we tend to naturally look at the negative things in life, but I challenge you to start looking for the positive. What things are you grateful for? One thing that has worked for me is to write 3 things I'm grateful for first thing in the morning. It helps me start my day off with a positive mindset. Give it a try and maybe that will work for you too.

You must be positive and enjoy the journey! That's why we celebrate the small wins because progress is progress. Smile and laugh more. Aside from everything that I mentioned in the book, laughter really is the best medicine. It is easier said than done, but it will help you get through the tough days so make sure you plan some fun time in your life. Remember if you fail to plan then you plan to fail. Are you planning your days to include healthy eating, good sleep, exercise and stress management? How can you prepare yourself to become more victorious?

One way I do it is through my daily planner. I schedule in the things that are most important for me to get done that day and it helps me see where my time is being spent. And spending at least 10 minutes a day to meditate can be a game changer in your life. We generally spend a lot of time worrying about trivial things with our mind fixed on the future, and we spend much less time actually focusing on being present. Believe it or not, research has shown that people who meditate have lower blood pressure, decreased stress levels and are overall more happy!

As I have mentioned before consistency is key. Do not ruminate or get hung up on any one bad day. The ultimate factor would be how consistent you have been for the weeks, months and years. Aim to consistently balance yourself in all areas. Dedication and commitment are very important as well. Achieving permanent weight loss and living a healthy fruitful life takes commitment and is not something you dabble your feet into.

Impartial effort gets impartial results. Remember that even though you may be committed and dedicated, you must also set your environment up for success because you can't always rely on your will power. Your environment must be set up for success for you to win. For example, is your pantry full of junk food? Do you have bags of sugar and candy in your cabinets? The secret is to remove all temptations right from the beginning!

WIN IN YOUR WELLNESS

Nutrition is by far the most important determinant of fat and weight loss. As you focus on improving your healthy eating habits you should also incorporate some resistance training during the week. If you are injured then speaking with a Physical Therapist will be the best person to advise you on what exercises you can perform. Note, just because you are injured it does not mean that you cannot exercise the other parts of your body. You need to know what exercises you can do and what exercises you should absolutely not do. For example, if you have a knee injury then it should be completely fine for you to perform upper body resistance training. Once again, I recommend you to speak with a Physical Therapist first. At the bare minimum, you should aim to at least get 30 minutes of movement or some type of exercise a day. A higher goal would be to exercise an hour a day for five days a week.

Resistance training or weight lifting should be done at least three times a week to help you build some lean muscle. The more you exercise the more calories you will burn and ultimately the more weight you will lose. You want to make sure you start slowly and gradually when first exercising. There are several health consequences from doing too much too soon such as rhabdomyolysis, which is a serious injury caused by damage to your muscle tissues. Do you see why it's important to speak with a Physical Therapist if you need help in creating an individualized exercise program?

The secret to exercising is to find an activity that you like and is really enjoyable to you. Nothing is worse than performing the same type of exercise and being bored with it because you know it's good for you. It's equivalent to eating a basic boring salad and chewing on it with disgust on your face because you know it's good for you as well. Kale me now! If you find an activity that is fun for you and you don't think of it as typical exercise, then the activity won't feel so much like a chore. It's more important that you have more movement in your life then to solely focus on the type of exercise when you are first starting. Just get in the good habit of moving! This can be a simple as taking a morning walk or predetermined evening walk right after dinner.

The higher the intensity of the exercise the more calories you will burn. In contrast, the lower the intensity of the exercise, the less calories you will burn. You have to see what your body is most comfortable with and how you can progressively challenge yourself without causing any harm. Adding in cardio days during the week is great for your heart health. As you age and move less, your body naturally becomes more deconditioned and starts to lose strength. Your muscle mass becomes smaller and you lose more bone density when you don't exercise. The more muscle you have on you the more fat your body can burn. So, what are some things that you can do to get some exercise in during the week? How can you create some time to exercise during the day to stay active and mobile? Write it on the calendar and plan it out!

TOO BLESSED TO STRESS

Aside from good nutrition and exercise, sleep and stress management are extremely important as well. Did you know that the more sleep you get the more weight you can lose? It's true! Most people do not consider how their sleep and stress could impact their weight loss efforts. Less sleep and more stress can significantly affect your appetite and throw your hormones out of whack. To get a little scientific, ghrelin is the hunger hormone in your body that tells your brain when to eat. If you don't get enough sleep the levels of ghrelin rise in your body making it think that it's hungry and increases your appetite. Leptin is the satiety hormone which is the exact opposite. Leptin basically tells your brain that you're full and regulates your appetite.

When you get enough sleep, you will have higher levels of leptin in your body and will therefore not feel as hungry during the day. Your body will then be able to burn more calories as the levels of leptin increase. That is why sleep is so important to your weight loss success. Are you getting adequate sleep each day? Are you planning for a good solid 6-8 hours of sleep each night? If you aren't then why not? Rest and recovery are very important to your overall health, especially as you increase your physical activity. When you're in physical therapy you are progressively stressing your body's tissues so that they become stronger and more resilient, and your body needs adequate rest time to help repair your body's tissues.

If you're increasing your activity levels and your exercises are becoming more intense, then you really need to factor in sleep time. Sleep and recovery are not only important for weight loss and muscle growth, but it is needed to acquire mental focus. I'm sure you've had your days where you could not focus and concentrate as well because of a restless night. Lack of sleep significantly reduces your body's ability to recover and perform any physical work, so you need to incorporate a good sleep schedule.

Getting a good night's rest has numerous mental and physical benefits. The quality of your sleep can impact your energy, mood, memory, stress levels, immune system, appetite, speed of recovery from injuries and overall health. This is something I address with all of my patients especially early on in the rehab process.

One easy way to optimize your sleep is to go to bed at the same time every day and wake up in the morning at the same time every day. This will allow your body's internal clock or circadian rhythm to stabilize and be at balance to help you feel more awake during the day. Having an irregular sleep schedule will cause you to "feel off" in terms of your energy levels, so having a regular routine is always the best.

Now let's talk about the different types of stress and how they impact you. There is good stress and there is bad stress. Certain levels of stress are necessary for you to experience in order for you to grow and become stronger. Exercising at a tolerable level is a good stress that is put on your body for it to become stronger. On the other hand, life stressors are the bad stress that most people deal with these days that have negative health consequences. It's important to know what stresses you out and how you deal with those stressful situations. Most people will find losing weight in itself to be stressful and as a result will not follow through with it because of how difficult it seems. That is why you need an attitude of gratitude! It will be extremely difficult for you to lose weight and burn any body fat if your body is in a constant state of stress. You're too blessed to stress!

Scientifically, too much stress on your body will cause an imbalance to your body's hormones. It will be almost impossible for you to become healthy and lose weight if you have excess stress hormones in your body.

Cortisol is your body's stress hormone that has many functions such as controlling blood sugar levels, reducing inflammation and regulating your metabolism. The problem occurs when there are excessive amounts of cortisol in your body because it can cause fatigue, high blood pressure, weakness and weight gain. Can you see how everything is interrelated? Exercise, good nutrition, meditation and sleep can all help reduce stress.

You will be fighting an uphill battle in your weight loss journey if everything is not taken into consideration. Are you aware of what stresses you out? Are you aware of your internal self-talk? If not, please take a moment to write a list of things that cause you the most stress. Creating awareness is the first step for you to induce change. Everybody in life deals with stress, but the secret is how you react to it! Have you ever gone out to eat or drink in reaction to a stressful event? Or have you excessively snacked and binged out on foods because you felt stressed?

Do you do this all the time? Changing your bad habits and reactions to stress will play a big role in winning in your wellness. Imagine how much weight you would put on if you went out to eat every single time you were stressed. Consuming something may temporarily change how you feel in that moment, but it won't change the reality. What bad activities do you currently perform when you're stressed? What good activities and habits can you implement when you feel stressed?

Stress in itself can harm you both mentally and physically. Stress can cause fatigue, muscle aches, headaches, digestive disorders, anxiety, depression, low productivity, and bad eating and sleeping patterns. Can you see the importance of controlling stress? Do you see how it can stray you away from your goals? It's not only about your weight. It's your overall wellness!

Try substituting your bad reactions to stress with good activities such as breathing, stretching, meditating, exercising, sleeping and healthy eating. Breathing and stretching are one of my favorite ways to reduce stress. They are very simple to do and can be performed anywhere! I have created a stretch break guide including 14 of the simplest and easiest stretches you can do on your own. Go to www.drwinsecrets.com to download my free stretch break guide. I recommend you do these stretches daily to help you reduce your overall stress.

Congratulations! You've just learned the winning secrets and now understand why it's so crucial for you to incorporate good nutrition, sleep, exercise and stress management in your life!

TAKE ACTION: PULL OUT A PAPER AND PEN

1. Write in your journal or on your calendar your plan to improve your sleep, exercise, nutrition and ways for you to reduce stress.

2. To keep track of your lifestyle patterns you can download the lifestyle journal at www.drwinsecrets.com .

CHAPTER 8
OPERATION FOUNTAIN OF YOUTH

This chapter is all about giving you the best eating tips to maintain that fountain of youth. I will discuss certain foods that you can include in your diet to help you look young and feel young. Have you ever seen someone who looked really young and then get shocked once you find out how old they really are? In contrast, have you ever seen someone who looked really old and then get astonished once you find out that they are really much younger than they look? I see this all the time and always are amazed of the older patients I've worked with whom have taken great care of themselves throughout their life. I've had 85-year-old patients who look at least 20 years younger whom have kept their health, youth, independence, and mobility. It is my only hope that the majority of America can achieve the same fruitful life at that age.

So, what's the secret in the differences between the two groups of people we discussed? We can certainly blame genes and the environment etc., but my aim is for you to focus on the things that you can control. In the end it all amounts to how you take care of yourself. Are your habitual actions in favor of increasing or decreasing your lifespan? If you are someone who does not exercise, does not get enough sleep, maintain high levels of stress, constantly eats junk foods, smokes and drinks alcohol daily then you are surely on a race to the death bed. All those factors negatively impact your health and will make you look much older than you really are. My goal is for you to be the exact opposite! If you regularly exercise, eat healthy, get adequate sleep and have low levels of stress then you surely will look much younger than you really are. We will talk about certain foods that you can include in your diet to help you improve your health, weight, maintain that fountain of youth and prevent yourself from chronic diseases.

SUPER YOU SUPPLEMENTS

Let's start off with some supplements that can make you feel super! This is all about supplements or foods to supplement your diet with to help keep you feeling young, looking young and improving your overall health. Although there may be some crossover, this is different than supplements to specifically improve your recovery from injury or performance during exercise. Remember that if you have a medical condition please consult your physician before taking supplements. This is not intended to be a substitute for medical advice. Although I recommend food first, a multivitamin is a good idea to take for your overall health. It can even be used as an "insurance policy" just in case you don't eat as good as you should on certain days. Research has shown that taking a multivitamin daily can improve your mood and wellbeing.

Coenzyme Q10 is an antioxidant that is heart protective and can provide energy to your cells. Not only does it lower inflammation and blood cholesterol levels, but it can be useful for those with certain diseases of muscles and high blood pressure. Vitamin C is a powerful antioxidant that will protect your immune system, boost your iron absorption and help repair your body tissues. You can't go wrong! You can find it high in certain foods such as broccoli, brussel sprouts, collard greens, kale, cabbage and strawberries.

Omega 3's fish oil will help protect your heart and brain so that you can really feel young in the long run. I hope you haven't forgotten the importance of Omega 3s as it is a great anti-inflammatory and can help prevent high blood pressure. Go to Chapter 3 if you need a refresher.

Melatonin is both an antioxidant and anti-inflammatory that is naturally occurring in the body. There are no harmful side effects. It can help you boost your immune system and be taken to improve your sleep if you feel you may have a restless night. The better sleep you get the more energized you'll feel! 60% of the America is deficient in magnesium and it is important for energy regulation.

Magnesium will help keep your muscles, nerves, bones and teeth strong and healthy. I recommend magnesium oxide or carbonate when taking in a supplement form. Magnesium can be found in high amounts in nuts, seeds, whole grains and dark chocolate. Keep in mind the calories when consuming foods for certain minerals or nutritional benefit. Eating loads of dark chocolate for the sake of having more magnesium in your body can cause you to gain more weight.

Selenium is a powerful antioxidant that is also known as the anticancer mineral. It is good for thyroid health and beneficial to take to boost your immune system. Again, it can be found very high in brazil nuts, oysters, and sunflower seeds. A powerful natural antioxidant is green tea. Consumed consistently over time, it can help boost your metabolism, burn more fat, improve your brain health and lower your risk of diseases. Green tea can increase your longevity. Black coffee is also a natural antioxidant that boosts your metabolic rate, improves your energy levels, alertness and brain function. It also has effects that can cause you to feel the jitters if you are not accustomed to drinking it. If you are someone who opts in for the fancy sugary high calorie coffee beverages I recommend you to substitute it for black coffee instead. Remember you have to train your taste to slim your waist!

Lastly, probiotics are highly beneficial to improve your digestive health as the majority of your immune system is located in the gut. Taking probiotics will boost your immune system by improving your good gut bacteria and can also prevent the incidence of infections. Probiotics can be taken in supplement form or can be eaten in a variety of different foods. I must warn you though. Some of the probiotic containing foods can really awaken your taste buds as they may require you to be slightly adventurous due to their acquired taste.

The more of the bad bacteria you have in your gut the harder it will be to lose weight.

You'll also have a higher risk of developing digestive problems, autoimmune conditions or other health conditions with a bad gut. This is why it's so important for you to include fermented foods in your diet that will improve your gut health. Kefir milk is a fermented milk drink that is similar to a yogurt drink, but has a blend of nutritional yeasts, milk protein and probiotics. It has a tart flavor and is loaded with health benefits such as improved digestion. You may even be able to drink this if you're lactose intolerant as the majority of people do not report symptoms. Just be aware of the sugar content as some products have included additional sugar to counteract its tart flavor. Also, speak with your physician first if you have a compromised immune system or autoimmune disease.

SUPER FOODS FOR THE GUT

Kombucha is a fermented tea that is also known as a functional beverage as it is created with a mix of yeasts and bacteria. It has a tart flavor as well with a fizz to it, but it can be a nutritious powerhouse for your microbiome or gut. There are different flavors available in many stores, but once again be aware of the added sugar content. Kimchi is a national dish of Korea that has gained lots of popularity. Kimchi is Korean fermented cabbage (cruciferous vegetable) that has a blend of ginger, garlic and spice added to it.

I love eating this Korean superfood as it is also loaded with gut healthy bacteria, vitamins and minerals. If you've never eaten kimchi before just be aware of its spiciness.

Sauerkraut is another type of fermented cabbage with many health benefits. It is found finely cut with a sour taste to it due to the lactic acid fermentation. Believe it or not sauerkraut has more lactobacillus bacteria than yogurt! This sour cabbage is popular in the Eastern European diet. I first discovered it when one of my Polish friends used to eat it all the time with his potatoes and kielbasa. It is an excellent source of probiotics and it is also high in Vitamin C.

Miso is made from fermented soybeans and it is used all over in Japanese cooking. It is made as a paste and can be found most popular in Japanese restaurants served as miso soup.

There are also miso dressings available that can be added to your salads. Another traditional Japanese food that is made from fermented soybeans is Natto, however it is pungent and requires a very acquired taste. The Japanese usually consume it over rice and with fish.

Tempeh is another fermented soybean, but it originates from Indonesia. It is a popular meat alternative with vegans and it is found in a firm, dense cake form. It is nutrient dense, high in fiber and protein with a nutty and earthy flavor to it. It is a probiotic rich food that can promote weight loss and improve your digestive health. It is a versatile food that can be made grilled, sautéed, fried, steamed or boiled.

Yogurt is one of the most widely known foods that contain probiotics, but by now you have discovered that there are more probiotic-rich foods available. When choosing yogurt be aware of the added sugar content. I recommend Greek yogurt as it is usually found with a thicker texture, more protein and less sugar. It is a wonderful snack that can help you feel fuller with less calories. It is higher in calcium and is an excellent option for older adults to help maintain their bone health. Try purchasing plain Greek yogurt and add your own choice of fruits to it.

Apple cider vinegar can also keep your gut healthy as it is great to add in salads and sauces. It can help regulate your blood sugar and promote weight loss when you substitute it for other food items. It can be used for many cooking purposes, even to naturally preserve your food. You can even add in a couple tablespoons into your glass of water. Although it has important health benefits, don't think of it as a "miracle" food. All the foods that I have listed can help improve your immune system and give you a healthy gut, but they aren't a "cure all" food.

By incorporating these foods into your diet, it will be easier to lose weight, but I recommend you to try them one at a time as they may require an acquired taste.

A common question that I hear all the time is "What foods can I eat to burn my belly fat?"

Although there aren't any specific foods that will instantly burn your body fat, there are foods that you can include in your diet to help promote it. Remember the winning secrets! You must not only take into consideration your nutrition, but you must also factor in the other areas in your life that can impact your health. Some healing "belly burning" foods that are more familiar to you are whey protein, cherries, peppers, bone broth, green tea, brussel sprouts, cabbage, broccoli, cauliflower and grapefruit. High protein, high fiber, nutrient dense and spicy foods have shown to impact your ability to burn more fat. Other foods to help you sustain that fountain of youth are the anti-inflammatory foods listed in Chapter 4.

Now I may have discussed some new foods that you may not have ever heard about or tried. It is time to take action upon the new information you have learned. Before you move on I would like for you to answer 5 questions and implement them. Remember, consistency is key!

TAKE ACTION: TRY SOMETHING NEW

1. What new foods will you try?

2. When will you incorporate the foods?

3. How will you incorporate the foods?

4. What new supplements can you incorporate?

    If you want to try a certain supplement I recommend that you talk to your physician or seek a qualified Registered Dietitian to confirm that it will be safe and effective for you. To find one now you can go to coach.drwinsecrets.com

CHAPTER 9
MASTERING MINDFULNESS

This chapter is all about mastering mindfulness. It is a way of eating and thinking so that you could be more mindful to what you're doing, instead of doing things out of pure habit. These are core principles that I recommend you incorporate in combination with the information you have learned up to this point. This is not about food labeling or calculating numbers at all. It has more to do with self-discovery and food freedom so that you do not have an unhealthy relationship with food. The first step in the process is to be aware of your thoughts and actions!

You want to start asking yourself questions when you're eating and really be aware of your thoughts. You want to stay positive and optimistic when achieving your goals with as much positive reinforcement that you can receive. If you truly believe in your goals and have it in the forefront of your mind it will guide your actions when eating. On the other hand, if your head is filled with negative thoughts making you think that you can never achieve your goals, the same will be true. "Whether you think you can or you can't, you're right!"- Henry Ford.

Be more aware of your thoughts and actions. Are you really doing what you said you were going to do at the beginning of the day or week?

Mastering mindfulness is a journey. It is not a quick fix! You may have to constantly reevaluate yourself to make sure you are being intuitive with your eating. I know I've said this many times, but it is always worth repeating. Think about progress and not perfection. What matters is that you are always continuing to make the right steps to improve your health and are staying in the right direction. Most people aim for perfection and that is why they get so discouraged when starting this journey. That only causes you to give up way too soon. Mastering mindfulness has many health benefits including reducing your overall stress.[1]

Remember it's not a sprint it's a marathon! Slow and steady wins the race. You want to have intelligent eating and be smart when you eat. Always think about having balanced meals! Yes, there will be times and occasions where your meals may not be so balanced, but that is not the majority of the time. What matters most is the consistency of your eating habits. You may have one good day or one "bad" day, but the big difference is in the amount of days that you have sustained a particular eating pattern. Don't shame yourself on one "bad" day. You must plan to win in your wellness! Consistently eating junk foods and going out for fast food every day is not intelligent eating.

THINK ABOUT EATING BETTER

You want to focus heavily on eating better foods and not only on losing weight. Constantly focusing on eating better has a positive spin to it and it gives you something to look forward to as opposed to losing weight. That may be a better metric to measure during your weight loss journey. Eating healthier nutrient dense meals will give you that small win to continue pushing forward as opposed to obsessively stepping on the scale. Instead of asking yourself "How many pounds can I lose this week?" you should maybe try asking yourself "How many healthy meals can I eat this week?". Do you see the difference?

You want to avoid distractions as much as possible when you're eating. You can easily become sidetracked and not be aware of the foods you're consuming when you have distractions around. I encourage you to have a good healthy relationship with food. One of the biggest reasons to master mindfulness is to learn how to eat foods that make your body feel good. Health is a mindset and is more than what you are putting in your mouth. How does the food smell? How does the food taste? How does the food make you feel? If you have distractions such as the television on when you're eating you won't be able to concentrate as well on your relationship with food. Having distractions around can easily cause you to overeat.

Having a food journal and actually using it can help you tremendously because it forces you to bring more awareness to yourself. I know I spoke about this before, but having one can help you stay on track. You will be able to physically see and write down if you are actually eating better or not. This takes the guessing out of the way. You will be able to see a better picture of your eating habits such as the time periods of when you eat. For example, you may realize that you snack on certain items when you are hungry or when you are stressed. This can really help you master mindfulness. The more often you can do this the more helpful it will be to you. As you can see this is not a diet to follow, but it is more of principles that you can take with you wherever you go.

Avoid diet mentality because it is such a short-term process. If there is a diet to follow I recommend the "Winning Diet", which is a healthy pattern of eating that works for you and that you can sustain in the long term. Part of a winning diet is for you to become aware of your thoughts, actions and to master mindfulness. You want to honor your hunger when you're hungry because your body is yearning for nutrients. A diet mentality may cause you to ignore your body's natural hunger signals and create an unhealthy relationship with food that can potentially develop into an eating disorder. Give yourself permission to eat, but think of intelligent eating. Do not think that you have to starve in order to lose weight.

"You are what you eat". Have you heard of the phrase before? It is certainly correct, but be careful to not misinterpret it. Your body will look and function at the capacity of the fuel you provide it with, but do not think that what you eat defines who you are. You are still able to lose weight while still having your favorite foods. You just have to account for it and understand these principles.

Be aware of your satiety level or how full you are. Most people overeat during their meals because they aren't paying attention to how full they are. Perhaps it's because of all the distractions or they just aren't truly paying attention. Or is it because they think they aren't full yet? You want to eat until the point where you are satisfied. You want to eat to the point where you feel satisfied enough and when it's not as necessary for you to eat more food. For example, if you wanted to eat more food you probably could, but you know you don't have to because you aren't so hungry anymore. This requires you to pay attention to how full you are. You don't have to stuff yourself with every meal when you're eating like it is Thanksgiving. Let's be honest, nobody pays attention to how full they are on Thanksgiving, but that's beside the point. On a scale from 1-10 (1 = starving, 10 = stomach on Thanksgiving) you want to eat when you feel you're at about a 7/10. Remember to eat slow because if you rush your meals you won't give your brain enough time to process the fact that you may be full.

Honor your health. Aim for longevity and not just aesthetics. We tend to do more for other people than for ourselves. If you need some extra motivation during this journey, think of people that matter to you most. Think of how many lives you impact. Think about how important you may be to other people's lives. This can be friends, family, colleagues, clients etc. Shifting your frame of mind to think that you are helping others around you more by continuing to honor your health can make a big difference. "Take care of your body it's the only place you have to live." - *Jim Rohn*

Be respectful of your body and your mind. Continuing to be aware of your thoughts and actions will help you make better health decisions every day. If you are being respectful of your body and your mind you will make better health choices and not just better food choices. This includes exercise, stress management, sleep and happiness, not just nutrition. Doing this will help you foster and develop a good relationship with food so that you won't feel guilty when eating. You will know how to balance yourself appropriately and will therefore will not feel bad when eating your favorite foods from time to time. I encourage you to take these tips to master mindfulness and implement it in your life.

TRAVELING TIDBITS

When you are traveling you are out of your element and your usual environment. Using the information you have learned to master mindfulness can help you navigate your way to succeed in these situations. Imagine how difficult it would be if you were following a strict meal plan or logging in every single calorie when you are traveling. To some this may be manageable when traveling domestically, but how about internationally? This can feel almost impossible to do! I will discuss some winning traveling tips that you can use anywhere in the world without driving yourself crazy. There are four keys to success in these situations, which I call the 4 P's.

You have a much higher chance of succeeding if you stick to the 4 P's, which is prepare, plan, principles, and proceed. When going on a trip you must prepare for it, both mentally and physically. Imagine if you were going to be traveling for three weeks right when you were picking up momentum during your weight loss journey. Are you going to just pause, stop and resume when you get back? No! You must first prepare for it mentally.

Ask yourself these questions:

1. How will I stay healthy?
2. What can I do to stick to my goals?
3. Can I master mindfulness?

Be honest with yourself and write your answers down. Preparation is key. Can you envision yourself staying healthy, sticking to your goals and mastering mindfulness during your trip? Next you must prepare yourself physically.

Ask yourself these questions:

1. How can I get exercise?
2. Can I make time to exercise?
3. What will I do to stay active?

After answering these questions, the next thing you have to do is plan for it. Remember that if you fail to plan then you plan to fail!

Ask yourself these questions:

1. What will I eat?
2. What do I want to eat?
3. Where will I go to eat?
4. What foods will I pack?
5. What foods will I buy?

6. When will I exercise?
7. Where will I exercise?
8. How often will I exercise?
9. How long will I exercise?
10. What types of exercise will I do?

You should be able to answer the questions above before you start your trip. Here are some ideas of foods to pack when traveling: granola bar, trail mix, fruit, nuts, sandwich, wraps, yogurt, milk, peanut butter, cheese, applesauce, instant oatmeal and beef jerky.

Principles to follow:

1. Keep an attitude of gratitude
2. Avoid diet mentality
3. Progress not perfection
4. Intelligent eating
5. Focus on eating better foods
6. Know when you're satisfied
7. Honor your health
8. Give yourself permission to eat
9. Satisfy your feelings without food
10. Ask yourself, am I hungry, bored or stressed?

After you have prepared, planned and reviewed the principles you may then proceed. You will now be better guided on what foods to choose and what foods to lose. If you're focused on making better food choices you can save yourself lots of extra unnecessary calories during your trip. For example, instead of burgers and fries maybe you can have a salad with chicken and sweet potato. Instead of creamy fettuccine alfredo maybe you can have shrimp pasta with tomato sauce? Instead of loaded nachos maybe you can have chicken fajitas? These are all simple examples of healthier alternatives or substitutions you can make.

Dr. Austin Win

TAKE ACTION: EAT OUT AND EAT HEALTHY

From the list below what things can you see yourself doing?
Please a check mark right next to the number

1. Snack on a fruit or vegetable before you arrive to a restaurant
2. Make special requests like sauces and dressings on the side
3. Order an appetizer and salad instead of an entree
4. Drink water with your meals
5. Share desserts
6. Take ½ your entree home by asking for a container before the food arrives
7. Skip the free order of rolls or add no fat to the rolls
8. Review menus online before you go
9. Choose a healthier restaurant
10. End your meals with a predetermined walk

CHAPTER 10
INJURED TO IN SHAPE

This chapter is all about taking you from ordinary to optimized as you pursue a fitness journey. As you continue to lose weight and ascend into fitness after an injury, there are concepts you must know to properly keep you fueled for your workouts. Sports nutrition can be complex, but my goal here is to give you simple and solid principles that you can follow. This will become more applicable as you graduate from physical therapy and return to sport or move on to higher intensity training. Optimizing your nutrition can improve your peak performance, endurance and energy overall. Improper nutrition during exercise can decrease your performance, cause fatigue, cramps, poor digestion, and breakdown your muscle tissue.

If you're someone who has struggled with being consistent with good nutrition please don't worry. Once again this is not a diet. I am simply giving you more information to help steer you in the right direction. The goal is to have you consistently make better food choices while developing the right habits so that you can feel your best and perform your best without traditional yo-yo dieting. We are going to discuss what to eat and when to eat around your exercise.

Eating properly before, during and after you exercise will make a big difference in your body. You will feel better and perform better as you optimize your nutrition around your training times. I will provide general guidelines on eating around exercise for you to implement. When preparing for an exercise session, you want to eat a solid meal at least 3-4 hours prior to the training. This pre-workout meal must consist of adequate carbohydrate, low fat and moderate protein for easy digestibility. You want to eat well tolerated foods so it may not be a good idea to try out a new food right before exercise. You should avoid high fiber or gas forming foods (beans) and spicy foods right before exercise as well.

The amount of food you eat will also depend on how intense your exercise session will be. If you intend on having an easy workout that does not require a lot of energy then you may not need as much fuel (food) prior to your training. However, if you plan on having an intense training session that will cause you to sweat, heart rate to skyrocket and muscles to "feel the burn" for hours then it may be a good idea to eat accordingly so that you are fueled properly for your workout.

Aim for low to moderate glycemic foods, which are preferred for recovery and maintenance. These foods have an advantage when eaten before exercise by providing a slow release source of glucose. In other words, they will help you sustain your energy and blood sugar levels longer. Low glycemic index foods consist of lentils, whole grains, all bran, dairy, yogurt, citrus fruits, apples, prunes, plums, grapefruit and green vegetables. Moderate glycemic index foods consist of brown rice, whole wheat bread, watermelon, mango, dates, kiwi, papaya, raisins, cantaloupe, pineapple, banana, corn, peas and beets. High glycemic index foods rapidly raise your blood sugar levels and are found in foods such as white rice, white bread, potatoes, corn flakes, sugars and sugary drinks. Right below are some pre workout meal ideas for you to get you started.

Pre-workout breakfast ideas:

1. Peanut butter and jelly sandwich with boiled egg
2. Fruit and yogurt smoothie
3. Oatmeal and banana

Pre-workout lunch ideas:

1. Lean turkey burger with small side salad
2. Turkey and swiss wrap with side of fruit
3. Low-fat tuna melt sandwich

If you're still feeling kind of hungry right before your workout you should drink water or have a piece of fruit like a banana. Have you ever experienced a time when you overate right before you went to exercise? I know I have and it's not a great feeling! You want to give your body some time to digest and do not want to feel stuffed right before you exercise. That's why it's important to eat something small. You want to keep the food inside your stomach, right?

Nutrition during exercise can improve your performance also and your strategy will all depend on your goals. If you're training for a certain event like a marathon then your nutrition plan will have to be more specific and individualized. On the other hand if you're training for a friendly soccer game your nutrition plan will look entirely different. I humbly ask you to consider working with a sports dietitian to help you best prepare for these events. You can find one at coach.drwinsecrets.com.

When you are participating in prolonged exercise you need to have a proper mix of fluids, electrolytes and carbohydrates. You need to drink adequate fluids to replace all your sweat losses. Have you ever experienced a muscle cramp? If so then you know it can be one of the most painful things on earth! Inadequate fluid intake when exercising can result in dehydration, cramping and other issues. You do not want that. Similarly, eating too much fiber during exercise can give you intestinal pains. You definitely don't want that either.

Water should be sufficient to hydrate you during exercise, however when having intense exercise bouts longer than an hour you can also consider the following items during exercise: chocolate milk, coconut water, juice, lemonade, fruit and sports bars. The purpose of maintaining hydration is to also replace electrolytes lost during sweating when exercising for long periods of time.

<u>Hydration guidelines:</u>

- Drink 1-2 cups water four hours prior to exercise
- Drink at least 1-2 cups of water every 30 min of exercise
- Drink 2-3 cups of water for every pound of body weight lost after exercise

Post-workout meals or recovery meals will help you minimize fatigue, prevent soreness and repair/build muscle tissue. It's important to eat right after your workout, ideally within an hr., to refuel and restore your energy through proper nutrition. You do not want to have a long window of time where you will eat after your workout. Try to avoid those large gaps of time by preparing for it. Start building the habit now. Choose a meal that is rich in protein with some complex carbohydrates (brown rice or quinoa) and vegetables. You can even add anti-inflammatory Omega 3's and some enzymatic foods such as fresh fruits after your exercise session. Another idea is to have a healthy protein shake to ensure you get some nutrients in after your workout if you don't have a meal prepared. Here are some ideas for you below.

<u>Post-workout meal ideas:</u>

1. Turkey, avocado and veggie whole grain sandwich
2. Brown rice with beans, tomatoes, veggies, chicken and avocado
3. Stir-fried chicken and veggies with sesame seeds and brown rice
4. Grilled salmon and broccoli with sweet or purple potatoes

To get a printout of eating to fuel for exercise you can go to www.drwinsecrets.com and download it there. If you are unable to cook or prepare your meals, then you must at least plan where you plan to eat your meals. To take it a step further you can plan exactly what you will eat after your workout and where. That will be the best way for you to make sure you stay on track. A lack of preparation will lead you to eat foods that you know will not benefit you. We all only have so much self-control until we give in to our indulgences. The point is that you will feed your habits and you do not always want to leave it up to self-control. Recognize your own patterns and eliminate the need to exercise self-control by not giving yourself too many options.

FOOD FIRST, SUPPLEMENTS SECOND

There are several ergogenic aids or sports supplements available that are used to enhance athletic performance. You already know that I always emphasize food first as I do not recommend you substituting supplements for whole nutritious foods. Once again, depending on your fitness goals there are a myriad of supplements that you can take to give you an edge. First off what are your goals? Are you a person who casually likes to exercise or are you an avid gym goer who wants to become an athlete?

Before consuming any supplements or ergogenic aids you must ask yourself if the supplement is safe, legal, ethical and effective. I always promote safety first! Do not take anything you don't understand and don't take advice from others who do not have the proper knowledge. It's important that you get advice from a physician or a qualified Registered Dietitian before taking any supplements.

Let's talk about some safe supplements that you can take to improve your athletic performance. Once again this is by no means extensive in any way, shape or form, but for starters it works. The best recommendation I can make is for you to work specifically with a sports dietitian who can best help you with your individualized needs. You can go to coach.drwinsecrets.com to find one that will best suit you.

Your protein needs are increased when you are performing higher intensity exercises and achieving fitness. Sometimes carrying whole foods may not be an option and whey protein may be an ideal way for you to supplement your protein intake. Whey protein is affordable, convenient, tasty and has the highest amount of leucine available, which is an essential amino acid. Athletes can require up to 2.0 g protein per kg of body weight, or 1g protein per lb. of body weight daily. For example, if you weigh 180 lbs. you may require 180g protein a day.

Creatine monohydrate is considered the most effective ergogenic aid in terms of increasing high-intensity exercise capacity and lean body mass during training. It is generally regarded as safe, and possibly beneficial in regard to preventing injury when taken within recommended guidelines. There is no scientific evidence that the short- or long-term use of creatine monohydrate has any detrimental effects on healthy individuals. Creatine monohydrate is found naturally in meats and fish. Ingesting small amounts of creatine monohydrate (2–3 g/d) will increase muscle creatine stores over a 3–4 week period. For optimal results, consume 0.3 grams/kg/day of creatine monohydrate for at least 3 days followed by 3–5 g/d thereafter to maintain elevated stores provide optimal results. Maintenance phase is approximately 5g/day.

Combining protein and creatine with regular resistance training can show greater improvements in your strength and body composition. Caffeine has also been shown to be effective as an ergogenic aid, as well as a stimulant to promote fat and weight loss. Research has shown that those who have ingested caffeine prior to exercise have displayed improved speed and power during their exercise activity. Caffeine, which is found in coffee and tea, has also been shown to improve endurance exercise capacity when consumed an hour before exercise. 5 mg/kg of body weight of caffeine is sufficient to provide beneficial effects, but take caution as excessive consumption can induce cardiac arrhythmias and make it difficult for you to sleep.

Once again, the amounts and type of supplements that you take all depend on your goals. If your goals are to maintain general fitness then maybe a couple of supplements will do like protein and creatine for example. However, the higher fitness goals you have the more supplements you may need to give you the edge you're looking for. There is definitely crossover between the supplements I have mentioned before, which goes to show you the many benefits they can have. I will mention just a few more supplements to keep things simple and actionable for you.

Sodium bicarbonate or baking soda is beneficial if you plan to pursue high intensity exercise such as sprinting or plyometrics. During high-intensity exercise you have an accumulation of acid and carbon dioxide in your muscles that make you become fatigued. You can delay the time until you become fatigued by ingesting some sodium bicarbonate one hour prior to exercise. You have to start slow and go low when you initiate this as some people have a difficult time tolerating it in the beginning due to gastrointestinal distress. An effective way to improve your endurance capacity with high-intensity exercise is to dissolve about 5 g of baking soda in a glass of water and drink it twice a day for about 5 days before your exercise session.

An additional muscle buffering supplement to help you reduce the time until you fatigue is beta alanine. Studies have shown that those who have consumed beta alanine have increased their exercise work capacity and increased their fatigue threshold. When resistance training, it has also been shown to improve your training volume by giving you the ability to perform increased repetitions when exercising, which will lead to more lean muscle mass.

Combining this with creatine supplementation can possibly even improve your performance even more. Consuming 3-4 g of beta alanine over a few weeks can show significant improvements in your endurance capacity.

In addition to the supplements above, I know I have mentioned a multivitamin, Omega 3 and Vitamin C a few times during this book. They are still a good idea to implement as your training frequency and intensity increases. A multivitamin will be a complement to a quality diet, but make sure it has 100% of the recommended dietary allowance (RDA) for vitamins and minerals. Omega 3's will help you with recovery as well as provide you with the brain and heart health benefits. Consume a minimum of 500 mg EPA and DHA daily. Taking Vitamin C will ensure that you maintain the health of your tendons, cartilage and connective tissue. I recommend consuming a minimum of 500 mg daily. Remember that it is a powerful antioxidant that can improve your immune system and increase the absorption of iron in your body.

Congratulations! I want to thank you sincerely for making it to the end of this book and sticking around with me. I hope you have learned tons of valuable information and that you have been able to take massive action to drastically change your life. Use this book as a resource to constantly revert back to whenever you need help. You now have the knowledge to really win in your wellness. I have done my best to provide you with information and strategies for you to succeed in your weight loss journey, but I know that information alone may not be enough for you to make serious long-term changes.

That is why I vetted the best of the best Registered Dietitians throughout the world, trained them in the nuances of Winning Wellness, and continually work with them as they work with their clients to grow their skills. My team will happily introduce you to a qualified Registered Dietitian who we believe will be a perfect match for you!

My team of Registered Dietitians are the food experts who can best provide you with a plan including your exact nutritional requirements, especially if your medical history may be more involved. You want to ensure that there are no food-drug or supplement interactions and also guarantee a solid plan that will work best for you. Whether this will be for coaching during your weight loss journey or for an optimized plan towards your injury recovery and fitness journey, our team can help. To find a Registered Dietitian that is best suited for your specific needs and situation visit coach.drwinsecrets.com to find one now.

I am wholeheartedly committed to your health, success and overall well-being. If you cannot find a Registered Dietitian that is best suited for your needs please contact me so that I can help you get your health back.

TAKE ACTION: LIVE WINNING WELLNESS

You can make a marked difference in someone else's life by recommending this book to them. My goal is to impact millions of people's lives and if this has helped you in any way my hope is for you to help someone else the same way this has helped you by recommending this book. Someone else's life may be forever altered with your help and without you they may never find it. So, I ask of you to please write down the names of five people you know that can benefit from receiving this book and recommend them a copy. Thank you for joining me on my mission and making a major impact in the lives of others.

Go to coach.drwinsecrets.com to see how we can help you!

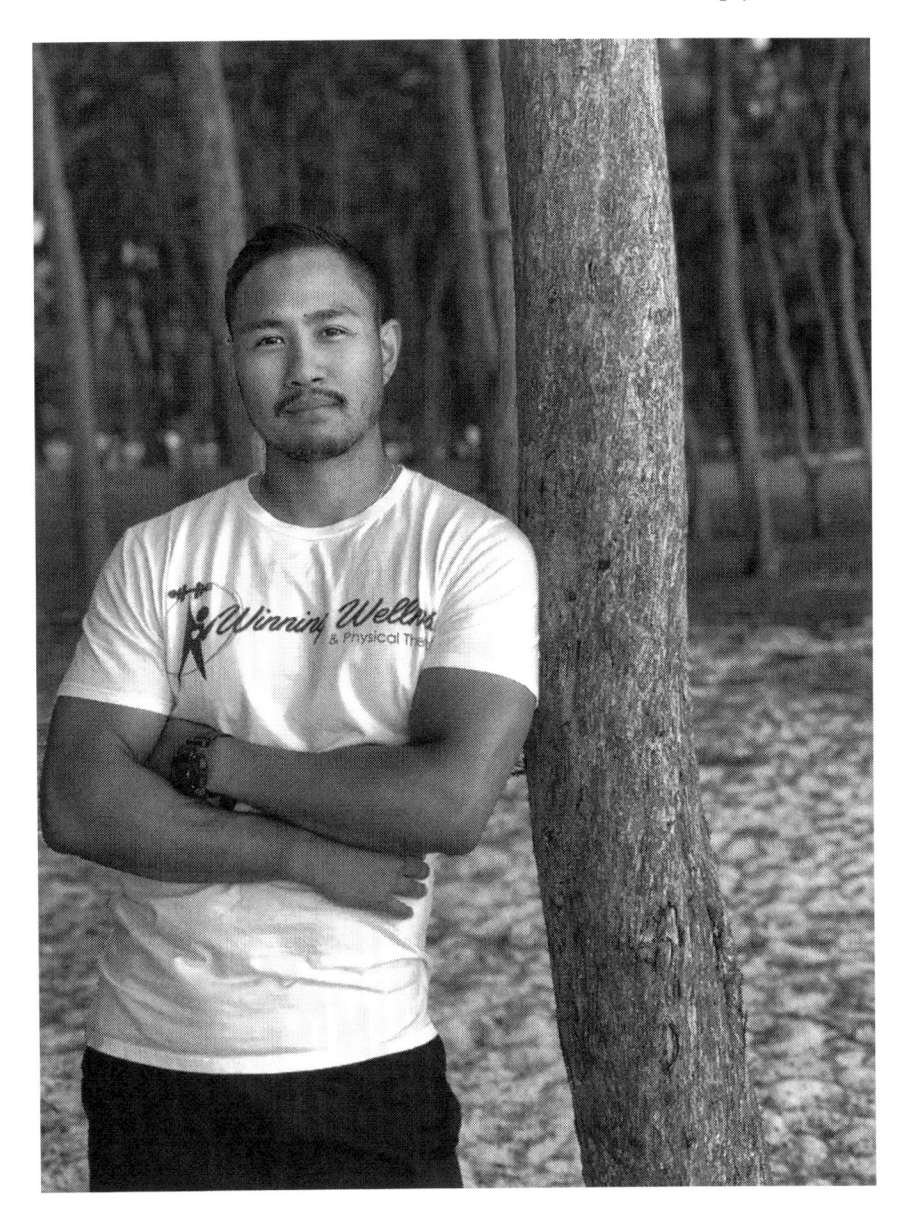

FAQS

Q1. What is a Registered Dietitian?

A Registered Dietitian (RD) is the food expert that helps people with their nutrition based upon their individual needs. They are professionally trained and licensed to help you with your nutrition goals, even if you have a medical condition or are taking medications. Working with a Registered Dietitian lets people live free from worry that their health is not in the hands of just anyone or a non-licensed "nutritionists".

Q2. How can a Registered Dietitian help me?

A Registered Dietitian can help you by giving you direct guidance for your health to make sure you are on the right track to meet your nutrition goals. A RD will help put to rest any nutrition misinformation you may have heard and guarantee that you will be on the right path to win in your wellness. A RD will provide you with full on support, guidance and any necessary tools to help you succeed.

Q3. Do I get personal support if I need it?

Yes. If you arrange to try a nutrition program with us, you'll be given almost unrestricted access to your own RD who will be on hand to take your call or reply to your emails, for as long as you need.

Q4. Does your nutrition program help someone like me?

Here's a list of the types of people our nutrition program helps:

- **People who want to lose weight, but don't want to crash diet- Why?**
  Because research has shown that those who continue to crash diet have higher chances of REGAINING their weight and MORE! We don't want that to happen to you.

- **Busy working people who want to keep up with their health BEFORE it's too late- Why?**
  Most people wait until it's too late to take care of their health. People need to be healthy at all times to continue to perform well in their jobs.

- **People who are determined to take charge of their health – Why?**
  Because those who are determined have the most progress and we are determined to help those who want to take charge of their health.

- **People who take their health very seriously- Why?**
  A lot of people who visit us are very "pro-active" about their health. That means they care about the foods they eat, health topics, nutrition, take vitamins and other supplements- and do their best to stay out of the hospital. They are very motivated to make sure they are fueled optimally for their physical activities.

- **People who are overwhelmed, stressed, feeling low on energy and confused on what to do for their health- Why?**
  Because most people these days are unsure of what to do or eat to take care of their health. They don't know where to start and as a result are lacking motivation, which are the reasons "why" to come see a RD like me.

- **People who are recovering from an injury…Why?**
  A lot of people don't understand how your nutrition can accelerate or SLOW down your healing. Many people want to speed up their

recovery process, which is why they often tell us they felt the need to try our nutrition program.

Q5. What happens if I start and I'm not happy at the end?

Within 30 days of starting I'd personally refund your payment back onto the card you've used – NO questions asked. Either you leave very HAPPY or you don't pay a dime.

Q6. Why shouldn't I just go and find help from someone else?

The truth is, many of the people out there giving nutrition advice is provided on the fly by anyone who is self-proclaimed to be a "nutritionist", without individual care and not licensed as a Registered Dietitian. It will usually involve you following a strict meal plan and going on a crash diet (as opposed to an individual approach where you don't give up your favorite foods). Putting your health at risk in the hands of an unqualified person can be dangerous.

Q7. Do I have to go on a diet to lose weight?

The short answer is no. Most people have a hard time losing weight because of all the diets they've tried in the past. The goal is to help you incorporate healthy habits and show you how you can lose weight WITHOUT feeling guilty or deprived from eating your favorite foods.

Q8. I'm confused on my diet. Should I go Paleo, Keto, Low carb or Low fat?

We do not encourage you to do anything that you cannot sustain or will do more harm to your body in the long run. The Ketogenic diet first began to help control seizures in people with epilepsy and other neurological diseases. We will help you to improve your eating habits and patterns, not prescribe you any one diet unless medically necessary. This is not another

FAD diet for weight loss. The goal is to ensure that you have a successful plan right from the beginning by creating successful ways for you to have a calorie deficit independent of whether or not it is low carb or low fat.[5]

Q9. Do I have to give up carbs?

You don't have to eliminate carbs from your diet. Most people fear that they have to give up their breads and favorite foods when going on a nutrition program, which is far from the truth. We will tell you all of that in the consultation.

Q10. What if I don't want to make another appointment after my first visit, do you take it personally?

Not at all and that's completely fine. Our first priority is to tell you what's going wrong and then tell you what you need to do next by drawing up a plan for you. Once we've done that and you're happy, then we're happy that we've given you full value for money.

Q11. How likely is it that your nutrition program will be able to help me?

If your problem or concern is one or more of the following areas:

- Weight Loss
- Energy Levels
- Recovery from An Injury
- Eating Habits
- Health Condition
- Muscle & Strength
- Performance
- Support & Accountability

Then it's 99% likely that our nutrition program will be able to help you out, and there are various ways we might do that.

Q12. Can I talk to a RD before I book just to confirm if this is right for me?

Absolutely. Just go to coach.drwinsecrets.com to request to talk to a RD

Q13. Will you do anything at the first session to help with my nutrition?

Yes. It's always our intention to start making progress right away, as well as help ease your other worries and concerns.

Q14. Will I get a meal plan or anything like that to keep?

You can get any tool that you feel will help you succeed. We don't think anyone should follow any specific meal plan for the rest of their life. You can only follow a meal plan for so long or under certain circumstances, but we will give you as many resources as possible for you to use and keep. We have plenty of healthy recipes and plans to get you started.

Q15. What will happen if I don't choose to go and see a Registered Dietitian?

You'll run the risk of doing unforeseen and untold metabolic damage if your body is not given proper nutrients in an individualized approach. A failure to start the right nutrition program could increase the risk of future weight gain, worsening in health condition, decrease in energy levels and performance. You do not want your current predicament to continue by not seeing a RD.

Q16. Is there another Registered Dietitian that I could see if I wanted?

Yes. We will always do our best to find a RD that we feel is a perfect match for you.

Q17. How long will it take for me to lose weight and get healthy again?

On average, from my professional experience, most real weight loss problems occur after failed attempts to successfully lose weight and keep it off after dieting. I encourage sustainable lifestyle changes, not recommending to lose > 2 lbs. a week, in order to permanently lose weight and burn body fat, not muscle. Our Registered Dietitians will be able to best determine what is an appropriate time frame for you to reach your goals when you start the nutrition program.

Q18. Somebody mentioned a nutritionist to me, what's the difference between a Registered Dietitian and a Nutritionist?

Every Registered Dietitian is a Nutritionist, but not every Nutritionist is a Registered Dietitian. To be brief, a Registered Dietitian has received the necessary education to safely and effectively help you with your nutritional needs. For example, when you have a tooth problem you go see the dentist, not a tooth specialist. If you have a health problem you go see the doctor, not a health coach. If you have a food and nutrition problem, seeing a RD will help you so much that you will not need to constantly keep going back to for the next meal plan or fad diet.

So, a RD will work out a plan for you to work on the actual problem so that you have long term results and not temporary changes. Depending on the state it can also be illegal for a nutritionist or other "health coach" to provide nutrition counseling, especially if you have a medical condition. Many good nutritionists or health coaches will refer their clients to RDs for the things they are not familiar with, such as diet medication interactions, medical conditions, recovery and weight loss.

Q19. I don't really need to lose weight per se- I just need some guidance to improve my eating habits and help with planning and preparing my meals. Should I still consider a Registered Dietitian?

You are PERFECT for a RD (and us). Some people think that all RDs do is weight loss- that's only ONE thing we do, but it isn't the BEST. The aim is to stop you from ever getting to the point where you feel slow and sluggish from gaining too much weight. The goal is for you to learn how to create smart healthy eating habits so that you are confident in planning and preparing your own meals, no matter where you are.

Q20. Can a Registered Dietitian help me if I have an injury?

Yes! A Registered Dietitian can very easily help you accelerate your recovery to speed up the healing process and manage the symptoms it causes. Many people come to a RD after having an injury (like during Physical Therapy) or are having pain inside their knee joints from the "wear and tear" (arthritis) of being overweight.

Q21. Is there anyone that a Registered Dietitian is NOT right for?

Yes. Anyone who is expecting a miracle and hoping to drastically lose weight very soon or have big changes after one session. Rarely possible without risking malnutrition, dehydration, electrolyte imbalances, metabolism shut down, muscular atrophy and other serious side effects.

Q22. I've been gaining more fat and weight around my belly. I can't seem to lose it and now I'm worried that I won't be able to fit in my clothes. Can a Registered Dietitian help someone like me?

Yes. It's a simple case of increasing your metabolism to get your body to burn more fat again. Most people restrict their calories so low that they'll literally starve…and so their metabolism is disrupted. A RD will give you hope and WILL let you and your metabolism get active again before it's too late.

Q23. I'm an athlete and I am unsure of what to do or eat to be at my very best. Do I need a Registered Dietitian?

Yes and Yes. You want to be at your optimal best as an athlete to not only feel the strongest, but to have enough energy to fuel yourself through your exercises to avoid sports injuries. It's the difference between fueling your vehicle at 87 regular to 93 PREMIUM octane. You will feel the difference after being coached from one of our Registered Dietitians, especially if you have plans for half marathons or other athletic events.

Q24. I don't have time. How am I supposed to do exercises AND make nutrition changes?

We hear this all the time. We don't expect you to completely change your life all at once, which is what most unqualified people try to have you do. After the consultation, we will come up with the best solution for you to be successful in exercising and eating healthy without feeling completely overwhelmed.

Q25. I know I don't eat that healthy. How can I make healthy food taste good?

Most people say they "hate" healthy food because they imagine themselves chewing on kale and broccoli or boring flavorless salads. The goal is for you to not feel that way and help provide you with healthier alternatives that you do find tastier to eat. Everyone has their own unique preferences and that is one of the things that will be discovered during your consultation.

Q26. Would a nutrition program help me with my pain?

Yes! Research shows that your diet can influence the amount of pain you may be experiencing. Most people experience unnecessary pain in their joints (back, hips, knees, ankles) because of the amount of extra pressure their weight is placing on their body.

Q27. Is a Registered Dietitian expensive?

Not in my humble opinion. It comes down to what you value, I guess. Most people will spend more each month on a fresh cup of coffee or eating out, than the "cost" of a Registered Dietitian who can actually save you money plus your health. And by the way- there is no set "price list". And that's because everything we offer is tailored to suit you, your needs and what you are hoping to achieve and even by which type of Registered Dietitian you'd prefer to see. Therefore, the "cost" to work with a RD at our place is based upon what you are wanting and hoping to achieve.

Q28. Do you have someone who specializes in ___X___?

(X is usually any one of these following areas)

- Weight Loss
- Injury Recovery
- Osteoporosis
- Fitness
- Heart Health
- Athletic Performance
- Digestive Disorders
- Allergies
- Autoimmune diseases
- Diabetes
- Pregnancy
- Oncology
- Pediatrics
- Geriatrics
- Renal disease
- Eating Disorders
- Women's Health

And the simple answer: Yes! We have someone who specializes in each of those areas.

Q29. Will starting a nutrition program with a Registered Dietitian help me heal faster?

Yes! You certainly won't improve your healing times by fueling your body with junk foods. The best time to start a nutrition plan is right when you're injured to speed up your healing and not waiting any longer to further delay the process. Waiting for a later time can only lower your chances of big improvements.

Q30. What does a nutrition consultation from a Registered Dietitian look like?

It consists of things such as reviewing your medical history, food and nutrition history, weight and exercise history, goals and creating a game plan. Ultimately our nutrition program will be tailored to your individual goals and needs as we hope to be the catalyst to your health journey. We do not believe in a one size fits all approach. Therefore, you will get the expert advice you need to help you reach your goals as safe and fast as possible.

Q31. Why can't I lose weight?

You are not in a calorie deficit. This is dependent upon your calorie intake and your energy expenditure. Note: If you have significantly decreased your calories (1,000 calories for example) and cannot lose weight, you may have disrupted your metabolism. Please speak with a qualified Registered Dietitian and do not lower your calories any further.

Q32. Will I get some tips that I can be doing at home to help myself reach my goals faster?

Absolutely! The goal is to help you in whichever way that we can. Primarily, we will be giving you the expert tips and advice from a qualified Registered Dietitian to "arm" you with the tools that you can use on your own to make a difference, but of course you need to implement the tips and recommendations we give you.

Q33. How long does a nutrition session last?

You can expect a nutrition consultation to be 45-60 minutes. Each follow up session thereafter is 15-30 minutes. Reality is, it will take as long as you need to get the help you came looking for.

Q34. Do you recommend supplementing my Physical Therapy with a custom nutrition program?

Yes! Take your injury as an opportunity to dial in proper nutrition while you're unable to do the things you love. This will allow you achieve your highest potential as you heal during Physical Therapy without slipping into unhealthy habits.

Q35. How important is nutrition to my recovery?

While battling back from an injury, the body needs to have the right ingredients to ensure optimal healing. Incorporating good nutrition under the guidance of a qualified RD can very easily accelerate your recovery to speed up the healing process when you're injured.

Your metabolism slows down with age and decreased activity levels, thus your body burns less calories than normal. By working with a qualified RD you can learn how to shift your eating habits so your setback does not leave you with unwanted weight gain.

If you are currently dealing with any of the problems mentioned and want further help or if you have any other questions please do not hesitate to email me at Austin@drwinsecrets.com

FREE HEALTHY GIFTS

($397 Value)

I have created a list of FREE healthy bonus gifts for you to get access to more in-depth information and tips on common nutrition topics. You can access all of the resources at www.drwinsecrets.com.

So the next best thing to do is to visit the website and leave your name and email address, then I'll know to send you some more helpful health advice like the ones you've enjoyed reading in this book.

- 2,000 Calorie Meal Plan
- Easy Anti-inflammatory Recipes
- Food Health Contract
- Healthy Eating Kickstart Calendar
- Healthy Grocery Shopping List
- High Protein Food Guide
- Kitchen Makeover List
- Lifestyle Pattern Journal
- Mini Cookbook from Registered Dietitians
- Nutrition Self-assessment Form
- Reading Food Labels
- Seasonal Fruits and Vegetables
- Sports Nutrition: Using Food for Fuel
- Stretch Break Guide
- Supplements for Injury Recovery
- Top 10 Anti-inflammatory Foods

REFERENCES

1. Grossman, Paul, et al. "Mindfulness-based stress reduction and health benefits: A meta-analysis." *Journal of psychosomatic research* 57.1 (2004): 35-43.
2. Lally, Phillippa, et al. "How are habits formed: Modeling habit formation in the real world." European journal of social psychology 40.6 (2010): 998-1009.
3. Flegal KM, Kruszon-Moran D, Carroll MD, Fryar CD, Ogden CL. Trends in obesity among adults in the United States, 2005 to 2014. *JAMA*. 2016;315(21):2284-2291.
4. Sacks, F. M., Bray, G. A., Carey, V. J., Smith, S. R., Ryan, D. H., Anton, S. D., … Williamson, D. A. (2009). Comparison of weight-loss diets with different compositions of fat, protein, and carbohydrates. *The New England journal of medicine*, *360*(9), 859–873. doi:10.1056/NEJMoa0804748
5. Gardner CD, Trepanowski JF, Del Gobbo LC, et al. Effect of Low-Fat vs Low-Carbohydrate Diet on 12-Month Weight Loss in Overweight Adults and the Association With Genotype Pattern or Insulin Secretion: The DIETFITS Randomized Clinical Trial. *JAMA*. 2018;319(7):667–679. doi:10.1001/jama.2018.0245
6. Campbell B, Kreider RB, Ziegenfuss T, La Bounty P, Roberts M, Burke D, et al. International society of sports nutrition position stand: protein and exercise. J Int Soc Sports Nutr. 2007;4:8.
7. Bucci, L. R. (1995). *Nutrition applied to injury rehabilitation and sports medicine*. Boca Raton: CRC Press.
8. Roland von Känel, Veronika Müller-Hartmannsgruber, Georgios Kokinogenis, Niklaus Egloff, Vitamin D and Central Hypersensitivity in Patients with Chronic Pain, Pain Medicine, Volume 15, Issue 9, September 2014, Pages 1609–1618, https://doi.org/10.1111/pme.12454
9. Dehghan M. (2015). Comparative effectiveness of B and e vitamins with diclofenac in reducing pain due to osteoarthritis of the knee. *Medical archives (Sarajevo, Bosnia and Herzegovina)*, *69*(2), 103–106. doi:10.5455/medarh.2015.69.103-106
10. Barros-Neto, J. A., Souza-Machado, A., Kraychete, D. C., Jesus, R. P., Cortes, M. L., Lima, M. D., … Menezes-Filho, J. A. (2016). Selenium and Zinc Status

[11] in Chronic Myofascial Pain: Serum and Erythrocyte Concentrations and Food Intake. *PloS one*, *11*(10), e0164302. doi:10.1371/journal.pone.0164302

[11] Felson DT, Zhang Y, Anthony JM, Naimark A, Anderson JJ. Weight Loss Reduces the Risk for Symptomatic Knee Osteoarthritis in Women: The Framingham Study. Ann Intern Med. 1992;116:535-539. Doi:10.7326/0003-4819-116-7-535

[12] Claire E Berryman, Sanjiv Agarwal, Harris R Lieberman, Victor L Fulgoni, Stefan M Pasiakos, Diets higher in animal and plant protein are associated with lower adiposity and do not impair kidney function in US adults, The American Journal of Clinical Nutrition, Volume 104, Issue 3, September 2016, Pages 743–749, https://doi.org/10.3945/ajcn.116.133819

[13] Dreyer, H. C., Strycker, L. A., Senesac, H. A., Hocker, A. D., Smolkowski, K., Shah, S. N., & Jewett, B. A. (2013). Essential amino acid supplementation in patients following total knee arthroplasty. *The Journal of clinical investigation*, *123*(11), 4654–4666. doi:10.1172/JCI70160

[14] Gregory Shaw, Ann Lee-Barthel, Megan LR Ross, Bing Wang, Keith Baar, Vitamin C–enriched gelatin supplementation before intermittent activity augments collagen synthesis, The American Journal of Clinical Nutrition, Volume 105, Issue 1, January 2017, Pages 136–143, https://doi.org/10.3945/ajcn.116.138594

[15] Raghupathi W, Raghupathi V. An Empirical Study of Chronic Diseases in the United States: A Visual Analytics Approach. *Int J Environ Res Public Health*. 2018;15(3):431. Published 2018 Mar 1. doi:10.3390/ijerph15030431

ABOUT THE AUTHOR

Dr. Austin Win is the founder of Winning Wellness & Physical Therapy and co-founder of Registered Dietitian Approved Inc, which is one of the largest social media platforms representing Registered Dietitians.

Austin attended Florida International University, where he received a Bachelor's degree in Dietetics & Nutrition with a minor in chemistry and psychology. During this time, he worked extensively in culinary arts as a Sushi Chef and opened his first restaurant with his family in Miami, Jasmine Sushi & Thai Cuisine.

After becoming a Registered Dietitian he went on to earn his Doctorate of Physical Therapy from his Alma Mater, Florida International University. After graduation, he continued to wear many hats as a Personal Trainer, Strength Coach, Registered Dietitian and Physical Therapist to address peoples' health and wellness needs, especially after an injury.

He continues to utilize his background in nutrition, fitness and physical therapy to inspire individuals to live more fulfilling lives through simple and effective wellness principles. His mission is to educate others to make better health choices by using food and movement as their medicine in order to prevent chronic diseases.

In his free time he enjoys cooking, eating, traveling, playing sports and doing martial arts. He also enjoys being a coach to young RDs and PTs all around the world.